S0-AYT-224

lives
in the
balance

BOOKS BY TILDA SHALOF

A NURSE'S STORY:
Life, Death, and In-Between in an Intensive Care Unit

THE MAKING OF A NURSE

CAMP NURSE:
My Adventures at Summer Camp

lives in the balance

Nurses' Stories from the ICU

Tilda Shalof, RN, BSCN, CNCC(c)

EDITOR

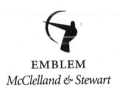

EMBLEM
McClelland & Stewart

This publication is designed to provide accurate and authoritative information in regard to the subject matter covered. It is sold with the understanding that the publisher is not engaged in rendering medical, nursing, or other professional service. If expert assistance is required, the services of a competent professional should be sought.

While the stories in *Lives in the Balance* are based on real events, names, places, and other identifying details have been changed for the sake of privacy and preserving anonymity of the characters.

Copyright © 2009 Kaplan, Inc.

Published simultaneously in the United States by Kaplan Publishing, a division of Kaplan Inc.

Emblem is an imprint of McClelland & Stewart Ltd.
Emblem and colophon are registered trademarks of McClelland & Stewart Ltd.

All rights reserved. The use of any part of this publication reproduced, transmitted in any form or by any means, electronic, mechanical, photocopying, recording, or otherwise, or stored in a retrieval system, without the prior written consent of the publisher – or, in case of photocopying or other reprographic copying, a licence from the Canadian Copyright Licensing Agency – is an infringement of the copyright law.

Library and Archives Canada Cataloguing in Publication

Lives in the balance : nurses' stories from the ICU / Tilda Shalof.

ISBN 978-0-7710-7982-5

1. Intensive care nursing–Anecdotes. 2. Nurses–Anecdotes. I. Shalof, Tilda

RT34.L58 2009   610.73092'2   C2009-901781-4

We acknowledge the financial support of the Government of Canada through the Book Publishing Industry Development Program and that of the Government of Ontario through the Ontario Media Development Corporation's Ontario Book Initiative. We further acknowledge the support of the Canada Council for the Arts and the Ontario Arts Council for our publishing program.

Printed and bound in Canada

This book is printed on acid-free paper that is 100% recycled, ancient-forest friendly (100% post-consumer recycled).

McClelland & Stewart Ltd.
75 Sherbourne Street
Toronto, Ontario
M5A 2P9
www.mcclelland.com

1   2   3   4   5   13   12   11   10   09

Contents

Introduction

In these 25 essays, critical care nurses reveal the fascinating world of the intensive care unit (ICU). Moment by moment, by day and by night, ICU nurses care for patients who have life-threatening illnesses or injuries. The stakes couldn't be higher.

In these pages, you will find stories of healing and recovery, along with others about decline and, ultimately, death. Some stories are about the period *in between* when, quite literally, lives hang in the balance. As they reflect on their experiences, these ICU nurse writers share their knowledge and expertise, as well as their thoughts and feelings, stresses, joys, and even moments of mirth. While their stories are all true, all contributors have taken great care to protect patient and family confidentiality. All names and identifying characteristics have been changed.

When it comes to writing about the ICU, Echo Heron was a trailblazer in her bestseller, *Intensive Care: The Story of a Nurse*. It is an honor to publish an excerpt from this classic, which inspired many nurses to choose to specialize in critical care.

The nurses in *Lives in the Balance* possess years of clinical experience in pediatric and adult care and a wealth of expertise in medical, surgical, cardiac, cardiovascular, trauma, and neurosurgical units. However, it's neither the population they serve, nor the medical specialty, that defines them. Critical care nurses share a readiness to take on challenges, a preference for fast-paced, action-packed work, and the courage to find ways to cope with tough, raw emotions that come with the territory.

Karen Higgins's enthusiasm for the ICU bursts from the page as she takes us step by step through the thinking process she uses to solve uniquely ICU problems. Mastering the ICU involves a steep learning curve, but Chris Kebbel took it on as a student nurse and then new graduate, eventually shaping a career that combines critical care with information technology. He recalls his early days in the ICU, as does Madeleine Mysko, who shares her first impressions of ICU nurses. Linda Lindeke recalls her career in pediatric critical care and the influence of a significant mentor.

Dropping down into Planet ICU as an outsider, Rosemary Kohr provides an objective impression of this rarified world, which she visits as a wound care consultant. And while the ICU is a place, it is also a way of delivering care to critically ill patients.

Sherrill Collings has to move fast from the ICU out to other parts of the hospital, and back again as she takes readers step by step through one extraordinary-ordinary ICU day. Kathy Haley and Janet Hale tell about the exciting development of Critical Care Rapid Response Teams. A cutting-edge technology to assist prospective lung transplant patients is reported on by Linda McCaughey. And if there was any doubt about the breadth and depth of nursing knowledge, coupled with the emotional maturity and communication skills that ICU nursing requires, read Meera Rampersad Kissondath's story. It is a picture of consummate ICU nursing.

ICU nurses know that our patients are not just the person in the bed. Families are often nearby, in need of information, comfort, reassurance, and above all, hope. Gina Rybolt shows this in her compact but telling story. Mary Malone-Ryan tells how she met the needs of one family as their father was dying. When patients are too ill to speak for themselves, families are often called upon to articulate their wishes. This situation presents Matt Castens with an unusual dilemma in his role as patient advocate.

In the ICU, death is an ever-present possibility. Sarah Burns tells an unsentimental but moving story of the end of one man's life. After Cecilia Fulton witnessed too many distressing end-of-life situations where her patients suffered deaths that were undignified and overly technologized, she made the decision to leave the ICU. As a community nurse, she helps patients articulate their advance directives and wishes for their end-of-life care.

The extreme suffering that ICU nurses witness takes its toll at times. As Claire Thomas and Elizabeth DiLuciano care for trauma victims, they show remarkable self-mastery in order to provide the best care possible to their patients. Bella Madeiros Manos bravely recalls an earlier stage in her career when the emotions her work evoked were just too great to handle.

The ICU presents particular challenges in getting to know our patients. Many are unconscious or intubated, thus hampering communication. When her patient becomes extubated and regains his voice, Sharon Reynolds discovers the person who had been temporarily hidden. Karen Klein learns about her patient through his wife's recollections. This essence of "patient-centered" care—of seeing the patient's perspective and attending to mind, body, and spirit—is conveyed succinctly in Judy Boychuk-Duchscher's ICU moment. Lisa Huntington and Bob Hicks offer surprising twists to "getting to know the patient" and the results are equally holistic—and humorous, too.

Entertaining, informative, uplifting, and moving, these stories show nurses who have found work to which they feel dedicated. Indeed, anyone who spends any time in the ICU, as either a patient or family member treated there, or as a professional who works there, knows that what is most *intensive* and *caring* about the ICU is the nursing care. Here are voices of ICU nurses.

Tilda Shalof, RN, BScN, CNCC (c)

Editor

lives
in the
balance

Intensive Care

~

Echo Heron, RN

THE LARGE INSTITUTIONAL CLOCK read 2:50 P.M., and somewhere in the middle of the eight flights of stairs, I wondered what I would have to do for the next nine hours of my life.

What would they need? Would it be simply a matter of controlling the pain with a little morphine and oxygen, or would I constantly be on the run, checking vital signs every five minutes, suctioning secretions to keep an airway clear, calculating drug dosages, calibrating machines, and listening to my sixth sense—all while keeping one step ahead. And, of course, a portion of my attention was reserved for the one fear that loomed larger than the rest, the one always present: Would I make a fatal mistake?

I reached the last step and had to juggle my brown paper lunch bag, oversized purse, and umbrella to open the door to the green waiting room. As I walked under the ACUTE CORONARY CARE sign, I noticed a woman with white hair sitting on the couch, crying. A younger woman with red hair leaned over her, touching the woman's shoulder, saying nothing.

It could mean something critical; it could be overreaction. But there wasn't the usual hysteria that came with overreaction. This was the kind of sorrow and fear that came from something tragic.

I opened the door leading into the world of the four fishbowl rooms, each holding a single blue bed for the critically ill. The monitor banks stood directly in front of me. Only one scope was lighted and running: bed two.

Before taking another step, I named the rhythm and knew what was wrong with the heart that generated it. Glancing at the assignment board, I saw bed two was mine.

I walked to my locker and took the blue cotton uniform from its hanger. As I slipped it over my head, I noticed an old bloodstain on the waistband that repeated laundering had not removed. I tried to remember the name of the patient who had contributed the small piece of color and felt guilty when I could not.

Next, my badge. I pinned the insignia of authority on the left shoulder seam of my uniform. RN, MICN, CCU, ER:

Registered Nurse, Mobile Intensive Care Nurse, Coronary Care Unit, Emergency Room. How many years of school and hard work did those initials stand for? Ten?

Lacing the white shoes, I allowed my mind to drift toward work. Bed two. How old? Man? Woman? How bad was it? The grieving white-haired woman in a green waiting room hinted at the answer.

Glancing at myself in the mirror, I hastily repinned several wild strands of my chestnut hair back into the knot at the top of my head and picked up my tools: stethoscope, packaged ointments, germ-killing swabs, and blunted bandage scissors. I was ready to face the evening.

The familiar subtle thrill began to well up inside me as I walked to the nurses' station. I compared the feeling to what it must be like walking on stage. Even though I had memorized my lines for the scene, no one ever really knew what was going to happen.

The report from Kelly, the on-duty nurse, was tedious and uninformative. That was unusual. Kelly was one of the coronary unit's better nurses, but tonight she lacked her normal enthusiastic energy.

"The patient is a sixty-eight-year-old male, admitted in the wee hours this morning. The diagnosis: possible cerebral hemorrhage. He had a head scan this morning, and I haven't heard results as yet," said Kelly. She sighed and leaned forward. "I just couldn't get into doing the job today, I'm sorry. I didn't bathe him, and I turned him only a few times and . . ." She took in a deep breath, then hunched her shoulders even more. Exhaling, she looked directly at me. "Jesus, it just seems so pointless. I don't like taking care of corpses. I just want to get out of here and go home to my kids."

I wrote down the clinical information about the patient without changing my expression or responding to Kelly's comment. We all knew the feeling of being forced to keep a patient alive long after it was determined the situation was hopeless. It was a futile battle that was more emotionally draining than almost any other nursing situation.

After arranging the facts by body systems, I looked them over once again and walked quietly into the glass-walled acute care room.

The rhythm of the respirator was in tune with the continuous hum of the building. The man's arms and legs were twitching, disturbing the plastic tubes that lay twisted across his naked chest and thighs.

I came close to the bed, which was cranked to the level of my waist, and looked at him carefully. With his slightly overweight, large-boned body, he filled the bed head to foot. A mist of sweat covered his balding head, and his skin was that particular gray color I knew well. The once-white adhesive tape, tightly wrapped in a thin strip around his mouth and cheeks, held a red-striped tube that invaded his airway and carried the warmed, moistened air from the respirator into his lungs.

I crossed the room again and pulled the solid blue curtain all the way around the glass, blocking the view of outsiders interested in watching.

Where to start? The mechanical assessment of the man's body was so like taking apart a dysfunctioning engine piece by piece. Neurological focal seizures; all signs absent; no responses—no one home. Kelly had termed it "vegetable soufflé." Cardiovascular: heart rate, 150; blood pressure, 80 palpable. Skin: cool, wet, and mottled. Color: bluish gray, dusky. Drugs: procainamide, dopamine, and lidocaine. Pushed through his veins by more pieces of mechanical apparatus, they did their job to keep his heart pumping smoothly.

I replayed Kelly's report in my head. He had been alive and laughing yesterday. There had been a special gathering of the family to honor him: Grandpa, Dad. I could see images of the silly predinner joking and the fumbling backyard football, then the after-dinner Grandpa stories he told, keeping the younger children entranced. It all had taken place fewer than 24 hours ago.

I saw the small, dried crystals of blood clinging to his nostril hairs and pictured the paramedics, their adrenaline running rampant, trying to push the tubes in without success. The man's broken ribs gave evidence of the prolonged cardiopulmonary resuscitation; so much effort without reward.

Spontaneously the seizures stopped, and I allowed the family in to be with him, one at a time.

His sister walked in first. Like him, she was large-boned. Seeing him, she made a half-waving sort of movement with her hand and laughed lightly while tears fell on her brother's arm. She stared at the place they had fallen but made no attempt to wipe them away. Without looking into his face, she shook her head and said in a very low voice, "Oh Colonel, Colonel, good-bye now, dear, bye-bye."

She noticed me moving about on the other side of the bed and started to explain. "I called him Colonel all his life. He liked it. It was his nickname."

The woman stole a quick glance at her brother's face and walked away from the bed as if to leave. With a jerky motion she turned back and started to say something to him, but her mouth moved without the sounds. Putting her hand to her lips, she backed out of the room, still speaking silent words to her brother.

I stood motionless until I heard the waiting room door shut. Coming close to him again, I put my hand on his and held it. It was moist and warm. With the digital thermometer I quickly took his temperature; the bright red numbers stopped at 105.2. From my training I recalled having read somewhere: "Anything over 105 is incompatible with life." Incompatible with life. Simple. To the point.

Ten minutes later a grandchild, a thin boy in his late teens, walked stiffly into the room. He stared straight ahead as if prepared to fight the enemy which held his grandfather. The boy reached out to touch the older man's face and caught himself. He would not make this real. This was his grandfather, a man he had loved all his life. He would not give him up to the world of these ugly tubes and sterile smells. His grandpa was the smell of pipe tobacco and apples. He was the tall, balding man always telling stories. Gramps was the wisest man he'd ever known; he would not let him go.

Suddenly his shoulders began to shake, and his angular face distorted with the shape of his pain. He turned away quickly and left the room without saying a word or making any sound.

I went to the bed again and looked at the man's face. As I leaned close to him, my hand moved to his forehead and slowly wiped away the sweat. I pulled the bloody tape away from his upper lip and was surprised to see the full white mustache. For a time I looked carefully at his face and decided it was a kind one.

Pulling back the lids of his eyes, I found large and unresponsive pupils surrounded by a ring of light blue. I moved close to his ear and whispered. "Colonel, I'm here, do you know that? I am right here."

Down at the end of the bed I massaged his purple feet as they lay still and ice-cold. I thought about his life, his work, and wondered if he'd ever gone fishing. "What kind of man were you really?" I asked aloud. While listening to the answers of silence, I noticed the monitor: heart rate 70; blood pressure 74. He was slowing down despite the drugs.

Twenty minutes passed, and the soft, whooshing noise from the respirator lulled me into a kind of trance as I did my charting and prepared the paperwork. A male voice startled me. Looking up, I saw a tall man with a middle-aged woman standing close to him. They looked worried and anxious.

"How's he doing?" the man asked, hope hanging on every word of the question.

"Not well," I answered. "He's very critical at this point."

The woman moved toward me slightly, wringing her hands. "Do you think he'll pull out of this? We've been his friends for so long. How long will he be in the hospital?"

I paused, staring directly at the woman. "He's not going to make it. His body is dying now . . . as we speak."

The man stepped toward me with a look that said he did not believe me; he wanted to bargain. "Look, if we go to San Francisco and hire the best specialists, that would help, wouldn't it?"

I stood up and approached them. "No. His brain is dead. He, the man, the person, really died last night; only his heart is beating and a machine is breathing for him. Not much else is functioning."

Both the man and the woman looked away from me, but not at each other. For a second I was afraid I'd said too much, too bluntly.

After a moment the man said, "Oh, dear God, I feel so bad." His eyes filled with tears, and the woman put her hand on his arm without looking at his face.

"He was very special, wasn't he?" I asked quietly.

There was a brief silence. Then the tall man answered me in a torrent of words that gained momentum as he spoke. "He was a wonderful man, the best of men. So intelligent, and boy, talk about a sense of humor!" The man threw his head back and laughed at the ceiling, though tears still dripped from his face. "He made everyone laugh. He tried to teach people how to feel good about their lives. He was a professor at Stanford, you know—very quick mind and yet always so gentle." He paused, then: "Special? Yes, he was definitely special."

The woman spoke up with a shaking voice. "Thank you, thank you so much for telling us the truth."

A lump came to my throat, and I could only respond with a smile. And with that they left me alone with my patient.

The thermometer now read less than 98.8 degrees. I felt the clamminess of his skin and had a half-formed thought of primitive things from the sea. I shuddered and walked to the outer door. Through the waiting room window I saw the white-haired woman still sitting on the couch. I opened the door and asked her to come in. It was her time to be with him.

She approached the bed very slowly, then touched his face and kissed him. "Papa? Papa, I love you so much. I always have, darling. Don't forget I love you so. I love you."

I pretended to rearrange the plastic tubes and gray monitor leads that were no longer of use. I was torn between curiosity and feeling intrusive, witnessing the years of love.

"During the night," the white-haired woman said, not taking her eyes off her husband, "he woke up several times, you know, the way we older people do, but the last time, when he walked back toward the bed, he called my name out. Just once. He looked so strange, lost really. Then he fell down, and I didn't know what to do. I was scared, and he wouldn't answer me, so I just kept talking to him, holding him, but he didn't say another word."

His wife opened her purse and took out an embroidered pink handkerchief and wet a tip of it with her saliva. With that she wiped away a smear of orange germicide from his chin. She picked up his cool, limp hand and put it softly to her cheek. "We were married forty-two years and loved each other every single day. He was my gift from God."

She stared down at him and kissed the palm of his hand. "I love you, my darling. Good-bye for now."

She put his hand down, closed her purse, and walked out of the room without saying another word. Forty-two years of loving and in one instant it was history.

Thirty minutes later, as I was turning him onto his side, I felt another presence in the room. Looking up, I saw Dr. Skinner staring at us from the door.

"The head scan showed massive hemorrhage. The largest I've ever seen. Stop all the drugs. The family wants it that way."

"Okay," I said, but didn't move toward the intravenous lines. He felt like an intruder, and I wanted him to leave.

After a second he said, "He was dead before he even hit the floor." It was his explanation, his excuse. He shrugged and walked away.

Carefully letting down the side rails, I gently put my hands under the Colonel's shoulders and spoke to him in a slow, measured whisper.

"Did you feel all this love here today? You can leave this behind you now. It's all right, I promise."

My face touched his. "I'll stay with you. I'll be right here."

A soft buzzing drifted through the room, demanding attention, as a small red light flashed in harmony to the sound. Blood pressure 40, heart rate 32. I squeezed his hands and felt a pressure rise in my throat. The blurring image of his face was changed and molded through my tears.

I turned to the pole holding the blue intravenous fluid, the one that kept his blood pressure up, and turned the plastic stopcock to the "off" position; then the yellow fluid, the one that kept his heart beating smoothly . . . off.

"All the pain is over for you now. Let it go. Let go."

His skin was almost white, and the ring of blue surrounding his pupils had disappeared, leaving only the gray-black window open to finality.

Again the monitor flashed and buzzed as the agonal rhythm, the rhythm of death, slowly snaked its way across the screen. . .right to left. Blood pressure. . .zero.

The respirator seemed suddenly loud and obnoxious, diminishing the dignity of death. With one smooth, swift movement, I pulled the plug from the wall, creating silence.

For just one moment I knew all the warmth and joy his spirit had ever given.

I removed all the tubes and tape from his body and washed him with the warm, soapy water reserved for the living. And as I bathed him, I softly hummed a lullaby, covered him with a clean, soft blanket, and said, "Goodbye, Colonel."

Just after midnight I walked through the empty waiting room, feeling drained. Yet, as I descended the eight flights of stairs and walked out of the hospital into to the crisp night air, I carried something with me. He had never spoken to me, there had been no gestures, I'd won no visible battles, but I had touched him, and his spirit. . .lingered.

Those ICU Nurses

~

Madeleine Mysko, RN, MA

It was 1969, and I was 23, a newly commissioned second lieutenant in the United States Army Nurse Corps. My orders were to report to the Institute of Surgical Research (ISR), Brooke Army Medical Center, in Fort Sam Houston, Texas. And I was filled with dread.

The war in Vietnam was going on and I was serving in the Army Nurse Corps. I was proud of my commission and had just emerged from six weeks of basic training. I was prepared to go to the battle zone, if that was where the army needed me to go.

The feeling of dread didn't arrive immediately. When I opened the orders and saw the words "Institute of Surgical Research," I had a vaguely pleasant picture in my head of a place gleaming with stainless steel, where one might don an immaculate white lab coat and take precise notes on a clipboard. Rather, the dread arrived when I learned that the other name for ISR was "The Burn Ward"—the unit to which the seriously wounded from all branches of the military were flown directly.

It wasn't that I was afraid of caring for burned patients. For that matter, I wasn't afraid of caring for any sort of trauma patients. I had completed my training in an urban Catholic hospital nursing school, where the Sisters of Mercy still held fast to the tradition that student nurses learned best by doing—and by doing a lot. Thanks to them, I'd had plenty of experience caring for really sick people, for the dying, and for the bodies of the dead. Moreover, after graduating, I'd held my own for a year on the evening shift in a busy emergency room.

It's hard to put my finger on the source of that dread. But looking back at the young woman I was then, and at the era I'd been trained in—a time when the nursing profession was undergoing rapid and dramatic change—I wonder if the dread had to do with the concept of intensive care nursing itself. To my way of thinking back then, an ICU was a closed-off space, crammed with scary machines and suffocating responsibilities. And the nurses whirling about at the center of those units were steely, a breed apart from the rest of us. I was only 23, but already I saw myself as belonging to an earlier era, to the breed of nurses comfortable putting their hands on the suffering patients, but not so comfortable with their hands on the ever-evolving, complicated machines that were used to keep those patients alive.

But orders being orders, there was nothing to do but report for duty. And so I climbed the steps of Brooke Army Medical Center in my crisp uniform and my spit-shined (literally) shoes.

The ornate facade of Brooke gave it a grand, old-world air—not at all how I imagined a modern "medical center" or a research "institute" would look. I walked through a cool, dark lobby with high ceilings and elaborate moldings. The polished floor squeaked underfoot, like the floors in the lobby of the old Mercy Hospital in old Baltimore, where I had trained, and where my aunts had trained, too. For a moment, it was like walking *backward* in time, not forward into the scary unknown. The dread lifted—but then I rode the elevator three floors up, to the Burn Ward.

My first impression of the Burn Ward is captured best in the incongruity I saw: the worn features of that old ward—the multipaned windows, the iron beds, the swabbed linoleum floors, the wooden wheelchairs lined up in the corridor, the antiquated bed-scale, the dark and cramped nurses' station—juxtaposed against the advanced level of critical care that the patients were so obviously receiving. Nurses and corpsmen hurried about that small space in their surgical gowns and masks, their mouths hidden, but not their eyes, which expressed absolute confidence.

The chief nurse, Colonel Katherine Galloway, gave me the tour. She must have sized me up immediately. She put her hand on my shoulder and said, "You'll be fine, dear. Don't be afraid to ask questions." The other nurses greeted me kindly, taking their masks off to smile and welcome me. The dread began to diminish. I saw that these good nurses would support me and teach me, and that I'd never be left to flail alone in a panic. And so I put on the gown and the mask and went to work beside them.

Blessedly, out on the main ward, there weren't a whole lot of machines to deal with. The everyday work was that of debridements in the Hubbard tanks, dressing changes, post-op care of skin grafts, OT, PT, and the continual stress of managing the pain. I learned how to care for burns. I was comfortable on the Burn Ward.

But at the heart of the Burn Ward there beat the vital sanctum—a space off the main ward that was further separated into two smaller chambers and closed off by solid doors. Beyond those doors lay the burned patients whose lives hung the most precariously in the balance. They called it the Cube (short for "cubicle"). In truth it was the real ICU within the intensive burn care unit. Every time one of those doors was propped open to allow a stretcher to go in or out, or to admit a long parade of doctors and visiting researchers on rounds, I would force myself to look in. All those respirators and monitors, intravenous lines, suction machines: I dreaded the day I'd be assigned to work in there.

As it turned out, I never did get assigned to the Cube, either because Colonel Galloway saw I wasn't ready, or because she never really needed me. ISR was blessed with a full staff of experienced nurses—more captains and majors than second lieutenants like me, a number of whom had served a tour in Vietnam, and a few who had additional training as flight nurses.

Still, every now and then I'd be asked to go into the Cube and assist. Looking back, I imagine this was Colonel Galloway's way of providing me with opportunities to learn at my own pace. I confess I didn't really take advantage of those opportunities, but rather became even more resistant to "intensive care." I didn't want to join the ones whose hands were always flying around in webs of intravenous lines, whose attentions were always riveted on readings, printouts, lab results, and the proper functioning of those respirators. I didn't want to cross over into what seemed to me a realm that was all about the intensiveness, and less and less about really caring. I had no ambition to assume the weighty responsibilities of "the steely ones."

One day I was in the Cube, helping Colonel Galloway and another nurse to care for a soldier who'd been burned over most of his body. He had just been returned to us from the tank room, and we were in the process of slathering Sulfamylon all over his entirely naked body. I remember that the soldier's face was so swollen it was nearly featureless. I don't remember all the details but with such devastating trauma, there must have been all sorts of things to manage for this patient: a tracheostomy, a ventilator, intravenous lines, gastric tube, Foley catheter. What I do remember—my heart squeezing in my chest even as I write this—is the enormous pity I felt for that poor young soldier, as I carefully applied the Sulfamylon. I also remember being relieved that that was all I had to do.

But there was Colonel Galloway—very much the nurse in charge, handling it all. She was explaining to the soldier what we were doing, acknowledging his need to know—whether or not there was the slightest indication he heard. Her voice was low and at the same time so beautifully powerful that even I was not afraid. I remember she reached down to the bottom of the linen cart to retrieve a single white facecloth. I remember that she placed it gravely over the soldier's burned and swollen privates. "There," she said, so kindly, leaning in to speak directly to her patient. "All done for now, Private Jones."

I remember it still, 40 years later: watching Colonel Galloway, learning that they are a great deal more than steely, the best of those ICU nurses.

What I Can't Hear

~

Judy Boychuk-Duchscher, RN, BSCN, MN, PhD

As CRAZY AS IT SOUNDS, this story is not an unusual representation of my daily life as a critical care nurse and clinical nursing educator in the cardiothoracic ICU at the Walter C. Mackenzie Health Sciences Centre in Edmonton, Alberta, Canada. In fact, as I think over the countless care situations I've experienced, which range from the absurdly humorous ("black humor") to the tragically heartbreaking, this one fits right in the middle.

Our unit routinely handles some of the most precarious of medical situations: instability of the heart, lungs, and vascular system. It is not uncommon to have VADS (Ventricular Assist Devices), balloon pumps, hemofiltration or dialysis machines, electrocardiographic monitoring, IV medication pumps, and various artificial ventilators providing a symphony of sounds, which only a highly qualified nursing ear can interpret.

On this fairly usual day, the crisis came early in the afternoon, which is when patients often are returned from the operating room to our recovery unit. The OR had called to update us on the progress of a pediatric case, a nine-year-old boy who was not doing well. The surgeons had performed a rather complex array of congenital repairs and the patient was expected to require fairly extensive support in the form of multiple inotropic, vasoactive, and volume-balancing intravenous medications that we used to regulate blood pressure, heart rate (and rhythm); high-frequency ventilation to maintain the patency of, and maximize the function of, his underdeveloped and now chronically damaged lungs; and ECMO (extra-corporeal membrane oxygenation) to ensure he had adequate levels of oxygen to sustain his life.

We had prepared the corner bed of our 12-bed unit for him, in an attempt to minimize the sounds of traffic around other patients' bedsides and to reduce the noise level his own medical interventions were producing. I can't say we were that successful—it was *loud* in that corner: transferring this patient from the operating room took at least 10 people including several pump technicians, 2 anesthesiologists, 1 operating room and 1 critical care nurse, 2 respiratory therapists, and the attending pediatric surgeon and her entourage of residents and fellows. As often happens during such situations, everyone was talking at once and several people had to yell their requests for medications or particular interventions so that they could be heard above the roar of the equipment and voices. One really has to marvel at the poetry of "nursing in action" that is evident in what we would call the "uneventful" transfer of an unstable patient.

And thus the "tipping point" that is the always-dangerous transfer of a critically ill patient was eventually replaced by the ordered chaos of an "admission." Those personnel not directly involved in the patient's care or in the ongoing monitoring of his assistive devices left, and those of us who remained were the ones charged with helping this vulnerable child on his long road of recovery. I had pulled slightly away from the bedside of this patient, returning to the nurses' station to get a different perspective of our progress . . . when I heard the voice. I couldn't figure out the exact location of the whisper, but realized it was becoming increasingly persistent.

Before a patient is transferred into our unit, it is common practice for us to ask the family members of all patients to leave the unit; we also close the curtains surrounding the other patients' beds to spare them any secondary anxiety. So the area was less crowded than it ordinarily is. I gingerly scoped out the area, trying to locate the source of this insistent voice. Then I located which curtain was hiding my anonymous whisperer. I poked my head through the drawn curtains to see a quite-elderly gentleman smiling at me, motioning with his hand for me to come closer and "shouting" in a whisper, "Nurse, nurse, come here, nurse." I smiled gently and entered his area, anticipating a need to debrief and reassure him about the new patient in the bed next to his. I took his wrinkled hand and leaned toward him. "Yes, Mr. C, what is it I can do for you?" I asked, fully expecting that he would need to be consoled and that I would likely be required to explain that what had happened to the patient next to him was not going to happen to him. But what he said (now shouting so that he could hear what he was saying) was, "Nurse, I just wanted to thank you." He patted my hand appreciatively and continued, "It is *so* quiet in here—I am having the best sleep I've had in years!"

I smiled, encouraged him to go right back to sleep, thought for a moment how rich my life was as a nurse, and went back to work.

My First Code Blue

~

Chris Kebbel, RN, BSCN

MY HEART WAS RACING. *What do I do? Do I remember?* Everything was a blur. All I knew was that the patient flatlined. *Asystole. Vital signs absent.* I climbed up onto the bed and planted my shaking knees right next to my patient's limp arm. I thrust my hand into the carotid, felt for a pulse . . . waited . . . The only pulse I could feel was my own. I positioned my hands over the patient's chest. *Have I landmarked correctly?* I tentatively pressed down. *The laboratory dummies I practiced on seem so inadequate now!* The patient's chest barely moved. Rob Fuerté, my ICU preceptor, came up beside me. He urged me to press harder. My heart pounded faster and my body felt electrified by the adrenaline racing through it. I pressed down harder. This time the patient's chest moved, but I felt it cracking under my hands. They'd taught us in school that you can break ribs, but I never imagined how unpleasant, how unsettling that would feel. I relaxed my muscles but definitely not my mind. I continued compressions.

Suddenly I realized my hands were wet. I could feel a soggy wetness through my gloves. I looked down and saw in horror that my patient's large intestine had been expelled from the wound over his abdominal cavity, by the force of my compressions. *Dehiscence—a splitting open of the wound.* I'd read about this in a textbook somewhere. Fluid was pouring out and along with each gush, long loops of large bowel. It seemed like I paused for only a moment to take in that shocking sight, but it must have been longer.

"Keep going," everyone shouted out, and I did.

That was the first time I participated in a cardiac arrest. Despite all my fears of doing something wrong, my patient actually made it, thanks to my efforts in this episode and the rest of his stay in the ICU.

I was still a nursing student when I helped save this patient's life. I was doing my final clinical placement in the ICU because I wanted to see whether, when I graduated from nursing school, critical care might be for me.

As a child I didn't plan on being a nurse. No young boy growing up in the 1970s would tell his grade school teacher that he wanted to be a nurse when he grew up. I hope that times have changed since then, but I suspect that they haven't.

In high school, I was a geek, and most of my teachers thought I would go into some aspect of the then-new and promising field of computers. However, I saw those machines only as tools. I wanted to stay with something more real and connected to people. I thought that forensics was my calling but after half a year in college, I learned that a lab bench was not where I wanted to be. I toyed with the idea of pharmacy or medicine but after talking with many people, especially family members who were nurses, I decided nursing made more sense.

When I entered nursing, my intention was to go into rural or outpost nursing. I had grown up on a farm and looked forward to returning to a more rural lifestyle after finishing school. After my first year of nursing school, however, I failed to find a summer job in the city, so I volunteered at the local hospital in the intensive care unit. My volunteer work quickly became a paying job as a ward clerk. I had the opportunity to view the expertise and compassion of the ICU nurses, doctors, respiratory therapists, and a host of other professionals. I quickly discovered that critical care nursing was what I wanted to eventually do. I continued to work in the ICU, first as a ward clerk and later as hospital assistant, actually getting involved with patient care. Each experience seemed to further show me that critical care was where I needed to be.

Working in the ICU has opened up many opportunities for me. It has presented me with some of the most challenging and amazing experiences of my life. I had an excellent preceptor in Rob Fuerté and the further luck of having a nurse manager, Maude Foss, who was open to the idea of having a student in the ICU, which was then a rarity (the prevailing belief at that time was that one should first acquire years of regular floor experience before graduating to the ICU). However, I knew exactly what I wanted. I was elated when, once I had graduated and become a nurse, Maude, who managed the ICU where I wanted to work, agreed to sponsor me to attend a critical care course and then to hire me, straight out of school.

I never expected the transition from student to nurse to be easy. There was an overwhelming amount to learn. During my first year, I was always lugging around at least three textbooks. I read most of them cover to cover, some a few times over. Surprisingly, the most challenging aspect of the transition was not my needing to acquire a tremendous amount of new knowledge or skill sets: rather, I encountered unexpected social pressures.

My being a new graduate caused quite a stir in my ICU. I didn't understand my coworkers' resistance to having a new grad working in the ICU. I heard whispers from coworkers whom I had grown to know and trust, now questioning the appropriateness of hiring me, a new graduate, straight out of school. There was this sense that you had to "do your time" in the trenches, aka the floors, before becoming part of the elite team in the ICU. I think some people were waiting for me to make a major error— and I knew they'd be ready to show me up when I did. I give great credit however to the many colleagues who did support me. This was especially true of my preceptor, Rob, and my manager, Maude. They defended me and at the same time found clinical experiences appropriate for me at every stage of my learning curve. They helped me succeed in a sometimes hostile environment. In time, the whispers of doubt, which had sometimes seemed to me a muted roar that would never go away, faded. The fatal error that some were expecting, thankfully, never happened. I moved into a full-time position. I started the standard line of 12-hour shifts, alternating between days and nights every two weeks. Eventually, I gained the trust and respect of my coworkers, and they won mine.

As the years went by. I was able to shift my focus from acquiring the practical knowledge and many technical skills of the ICU, to learning about my patients' emotional and spiritual needs, and to those of their families.

In the ICU, we see patients and families at some of the worst times of their lives. We help them understand what is going on and support them as they make some complex decisions and deal with some difficult outcomes.

Today, I am at a point in my career where I split my time between bedside practice and my medical/nursing informatics business. Many people told me that I would not be able to do both—each requires such a different skill set. I've managed to do both for over five years now. Being both clinical and technical is an ideal work arrangement for me. It allows me to identify problems in the workplace and to come up with solutions that others may not see. To my mind, I've got the best of both worlds.

Stranger in a Strange Land

~

Rosemary Kohr, RN, BScN, MScN, *ACNP, PhD*

THE ICU IS NOT MY "HOME"—it's not the place where I work—but I'm called there frequently in my role as a wound care specialist. The ICU is a world apart from the rest of the hospital. It's closed off by doors marked "Hospital Personnel Only" on one end, and at the other, a long counter where the receptionist sits like a gatekeeper, controlling the flow of family and other visitors. I use my identity badge to swipe the lock and walk through to the back entrance of the ICU, away from the waiting room with its televisions, aquarium, and anxious families who look up each time a staff member walks past. I rarely get more than a glance because I'm clearly not an ICU staff

31

member—I'm not dressed in OR greens or even in a uniform, just my ordinary clothes.

But I am there when a patient needs my services. I don't like to say "Doctor" because then some people think I'm a physician; I'm not, but I do have a PhD, as a nurse who specializes in the care and management of wounds.

The ICU is both noisy and quiet. When you walk in, the sounds of the machines coming from each of the bays where there are patients is very loud, almost an assault on the ears. However, the voices of the patients are noticeably absent: most are unconscious or much too sick even to be fully aware of their surroundings, much less to speak. In the ICU, each patient is in a large room, with curtained, sliding glass doors. Outside the room, nurses can sit and observe the patient while also keeping an eye on the monitors in the room. The ICU beds are high-tech. They can be raised or lowered, can pulsate or float the patient, and even transform into a chair. The machines whirl and beep and the monitors have colored screens covered with numbers, lines, graphs, and words. Attached to each patient are tubing and lines connected from the machines to the patient's fingers, toes, throat, chest, urethra, rectum, nose, mouth, and head. The patients lie in the beds, at the center of this little universe of busyness, often sedated, sometimes partially awake. Their eyes are closed or flutter open. They look around sometimes as a voice speaks to them, or when a hand touches them, or when a machine beeps, all in response to the ever-changing stimuli around them.

Each nurse cares for one patient, or sometimes two, depending on the complexity of the patient's needs or staffing conditions. The charts are outside the room and the nurses, when not dealing with the countless demands of the machines, or attending to their patients, often sit to record their observations, all the while keeping a close eye on their patient and the ones in the surrounding rooms. This vantage point, outside the patient's room, allows them to observe and respond quickly if a patient develops problems, or if one of the other nurses, doctors, or respiratory therapists needs another pair of hands, another set of eyes, or their expertise.

This is not my usual world and it is way outside of my comfort zone. It is far more machine-oriented and more spacious than where I usually spend my time, in the general medical and surgical floors in the rest of the hospital. To me, the ICU seems overwhelming, with its machines and technology. It is a much more sterile environment than the wards where I usually work. It is scrubbed clean. The tile floors are shiny, the walls a soft yellow, and the lights bright; it seems like an alert, active place.

I come to the ICU as a visitor, a consultant, to offer something specific, something they need. Many critically ill patients have wounds, either due to trauma, infectious disease processes, or skin breakdown related to a multitude of causes. The staff needs my assistance and my skill in treating these complicated cases.

"Oh, thank God you're here," says the nurse who paged me. She's enfolded in a yellow isolation gown that looks far too big on her. "We have no idea how to handle this wound . . ."

She sighs, and waits while I leaf through the patient's chart, wash my hands, gown, and glove. MRSA, or methicillin-resistant Staphylococcus aureus, is a common organism in most hospitals these days. It is one of the new superbugs that is easily transmitted and very difficult to treat. We do everything we can to fight its spread and I am careful to maintain the protocols to decrease its spread. Patients have died from MRSA and wounds are often MRSA's point of entry. As nurses, we seem to be in a perpetual state of hand-washing. Whenever I see a hand-wash dispenser, I automatically wash my hands—it's a reflex. I change my gloves almost as often. I wear no jewelry on my hands, not even my wedding ring, as the cracks and crevices are potential hiding places for infectious material.

Mr. Mountain, the patient I've been called to consult upon, is indeed a mountain of a man. At least, that's what I see from the doorway. The bedclothes are in a huge pile over his prone body. Tubes are everywhere; machines beep and whirl. I'm eager to get closer, to touch his skin, to see the flesh, especially the wounded parts, and try to fix them. As I approach, I see that the exposed skin on his face and hands is pale and puffy, soft and squishy like marshmallows. His eyes are closed; he has a tube in his nose and more tubes coming out from under the bed covers. The bed whirls and the mattress seems to be breathing along with him as it automatically adjusts to his body's position. I look closely and see that he is breathing little shallow breaths that move the blankets slightly across the vast expanse of his belly and chest.

I am never certain what to expect with wounds. Even when I'm given information ahead of time, it's never enough: I have to see it with my own eyes. Often, when I take off the dressing, roll the patient over if necessary, and expose the wound, it is very different from what I've been told to expect. I have seen some wounds that are truly horrific and would be beyond most people's ability to describe. But I need to put my hand in them; see down to bone if it is deep; touch, and see fluid moving, rivulets of pus when I press. I even need to smell the wound: that helps me know what kind of infectious organism is lurking. I know for many people, even nurses who are accustomed to dealing with the most intimate of body parts, some wounds are difficult to face and elicit a visceral repulsion. I think my own neutral, or even fascinated, response to wounds comes from my lifelong interest in art. When I was taking drawing lessons and learning to see as an artist, my "eye" was trained to see what was before me; I learned to record what I observed without attributing an emotional response to it.

There's another way I look at wounds. To me, wounds are like enticing presents: there's always a sense of excitement when you receive one, they are always wrapped up (in gauze and tape), and you never know what you'll find inside! For example, the dressing might be huge and the wound very small and insignificant. Sometimes it is deep and dark like a cave, the end point disappearing out of sight. There are often surprises contained within those packages. . . .

So, Mr. Mountain, where is your wound?

I ask Donna, the nurse who is his primary caregiver today, to show me. He was admitted to the ICU from home. He'd had a sudden decrease in his level of consciousness at home and hypotension—a severe drop in his blood pressure. The diagnosis of urosepsis, a blood-borne infection from urinary tract bacteria, was made. He is now critically ill and on full life support. Due to his overwhelming infection, the medications he's received, and his poor cardiovascular condition, his body has reacted by pushing fluids out into the tissues.

Donna points out some of the relevant lab work that helps to explain the leaky condition of his skin. His infection, despite IV antibiotics for the past several days, has not yet resolved. Donna fills me in on his baseline health, other co-morbidities, and his family's concerns.

Some consultants come in to see patients, never speak to the nurses or anyone else, write their notes and orders, and leave. However, I always see these consults as an opportunity to teach and learn. I like to discuss the situation with the nurse, include the patient and family if they're able, and also include the physiotherapist, the occupational therapist, dietitian, and attending physician, when they are available. ICU patients are usually in such complex situations that it takes a team to care for them. I enjoy this collaborative aspect of the ICU. It's a great time to share information, thoughts, learn something new. We develop a plan of care that addresses all the components of the patient's world—what it takes to nurture and heal, when possible, and when not, to care and comfort. This collegial, caring approach makes me think of Johnny Appleseed (one of my heroes, I must admit), who traveled across the midwestern United States in the early 1800s. His real name was John Chapman; he got people to plant apple trees, and he showed them how to grow and nurture those trees in orchards. Perhaps his story speaks to me so much, even today, because I grew up on a piece of land that had 36 apple trees, vestiges of an ancient orchard in my backyard, that my parents cherished.

We pull back the covers. Mr. Mountain has had a reaction to the drugs he's received that has caused further swelling with fluid. His body is covered in huge blisters, some still filled with fluid, some flat and crumpled with dead skin across his back, shoulders, and thighs. The skin, where the tissue has died and rolled off, glistens. There is bloody drainage on the sheets and he's oozing pink-tinged fluid as we gently move him onto his side. He groans, and his eyelids open and close.

My heart sinks. Even with all my experience, the sight of wounds this massive still stops me in my tracks. I will have to call on all that I have learned and experienced as a wound care specialist. What to do? This is not just one wound: it's many, covering huge parts of his massive body. He's not a small person to begin with, and now, he's puffed up like the Michelin man. My mind goes into a clicking, autopilot checklist as I scan his body with my eyes, touch his skin, and assess the edema and the circulation. Pain? Under control, thank goodness. Pressure relief? Appropriate bed surface: yes, that's standard for the ICU, which is a huge advantage here.

I think about what to do, what to do now. There is no simple solution. We can't wrap all of his wounds because too many parts of him need dressings, but if we can protect the newly exposed tissues, deal with the drainage and the blisters sloshing with fluid, maybe we can promote the healing process. . . .

As I think through my plan, I'm talking with Donna. We are standing close together, our long yellow gowns flowing into each other. Our purple latex-free gloves are tight, to maximize the intentionality of our touch. We follow the research-based, best-practice guidelines on treating these types of wounds and talk about the current research. For example, there are two sides to the argument "to pop or not to pop" water blisters. I am in favor of controlled removal of fluid in blisters—if there is a lot of fluid and, for example, if the blister is on a pressure point (e.g., the heel), preventing the person from walking. I ask Donna what she thinks; at first she is skeptical about my position, but she agrees once I tell her of the scientific evidence.

"As long as I can see why it's being done, that there's a good reason," she says to me as we gather our supplies.

Donna is right. As nurses, we have to be able to know the rationale for our actions, to be sure we are in fact "doing the right thing." I'm glad she understands the reasoning for this procedure; she can answer questions from other members of the team who might ask why we're opening these blisters. Knowledge is a powerful tool that not only strengthens us as nurses but also enables us to advocate for our patients and their families.

We gather the supplies we need—sterile drapes, a sterile scalpel, surgical gloves, and lots of gauze and pads—and set about treating Mr. Mountain's huge blisters. While this is not within everyone's scope of practice, I have the knowledge, experience, and judgment to do this procedure. I know I can do it properly and safely.

Donna and I work side by side, carefully and quietly.

She holds the gauze 4 x 4s to catch the drainage as I create the incisions in the devitalized tissue. As we're doing this, I'm thinking about what to put over these, to protect the skin. In the end, we decide to lay soft, silicone mesh over the worst parts and cover them with big abdominal pads. The contact layer can stay on for up to a week, and we can just replace the abdominal pads as they become saturated. Mr. Mountain isn't moving much, so we don't need to use tape. We wrap his arms and legs with a soft, non-woven wrap and then put stockinette over them to keep the coverings from riding up or falling off.

"Now you really do look like the Michelin man," I say to the patient (who still has shown few other reactions besides groaning and moving his eyelids). But I feel better to see him neatly wrapped. There's no bloody drainage on the sheets or the dressings. Things are neat and tidy—at least, as much as possible. When his family comes to visit, he'll look better to them, I'm sure. Donna and I appraise our handiwork and smile at each other: a job well done.

As I sit outside the room, writing up my notes, one of the other nurses comes up to me and says, "While you're here . . . would you mind taking a look at my patient?"

"Sure" I say, "just give me a minute to finish this."

I love what I do. I'm a needed resource, there to help patients, their families, and the ICU staff grow and develop. As I see it, the more apple trees, the better.

Discernible Markings

~

Claire Thomas, RN, BSCN

IT WAS A FRIDAY NIGHT and I was a little late arriving to work. I rushed to my assigned room and found an empty bed: this is an ominous sign in a trauma unit. I had worked in intensive care for six years, but only two in trauma; I was still considerably green. I set up the room to ensure it was well stocked and well equipped, prepared for anything from gunshot wounds to a motor vehicle crash.

The notion of not knowing the night's fate is always daunting. This empty bed would soon be filled by someone with a specific, serious situation. Everyone in ICU knows that feeling of being nervous yet simultaneously mentally preparing for a plethora of possible admissions, but few of us discuss it. Personally, I refrain from talking about it because, although I have chosen this profession and often thrive on the excitement and adrenaline rush, I'm aware that for the patients and their families, our meeting signifies the worst of all possible circumstances.

When I was satisfied that my room was ready, I made a round of the ICU to see whether any of my colleagues could use a hand—or more accurately, to socialize and to distract myself.

Not even an hour had passed when the charge nurse informed me that a multi-trauma victim was en route to the hospital. A pedestrian, in her mid-thirties, had been struck in a hit-and-run accident. So far, that was all we knew. Still nameless, "Jane Doe" was being admitted through Emergency, where our ICU's medical resident had been sent to perform a quick assessment. I was sent to meet them in CT scan with the bed. The victim had been intubated on the scene and several large-bore IVs had been started, but I knew they wouldn't be enough. After such a massive trauma, she would need resuscitation with large amounts of fluid, so we would need to put in a central line in order to access a main vein. We could see that she had lost a huge amount of blood, and she was likely bleeding internally, too.

As I received a brief verbal report from the attending physician about the patient's visible injuries, I watched over the radiology technician's shoulder to view the internal injuries of my patient on the screen. The picture was bleak. There was a small right hematoma in the parietal lobe of the brain, but no noticeable shift; a fractured mandible (jawbone), multiple rib fractures, causing a right hemopneumothorax, which is an accumulation of blood and/or air in the pleural cavity; a likely liver laceration; a pelvic fracture; and left tibia and fibula fractures. We would know more once we received the final report from the radiologist. My immediate concern, however, was that my patient's vital signs were worsening: her heart rate was increasing, blood pressure decreasing—she was intravascularly dry.

We rushed her up to ICU and into my assigned bed space. My colleagues, the other critical care nurses, freed themselves to come over and help. We had so much to do to stabilize the patient that none of us had even a moment to consider the tragedy or the person who lay before us. I delegated assignments. One nurse connected the patient to the cardiac monitor while another began setting up IVs and priming meds. Two others worked on the patient directly, cleaning her wounds and applying dressings. The respiratory therapist (RT) connected her to the ventilator while I drew blood samples. Someone called the blood bank to advise their staff that we needed a lot of products, stat. The attending inserted an arterial line and was preparing to insert a central line when the thoracic surgeon on call arrived to see whether his specialized skills were needed.

My patient's vital signs were still labile. I gave her Pentaspan, a volume expander, as well as normal saline boluses, one after another. I knew that I would have to keep on top of her fluid requirements all night. I initiated Levophed, a potent inotrope, in order to maintain her blood pressure. She was barely alive. I think we were all afraid we would lose her, but we couldn't stop to allow our minds to go there.

The surgeon decided to insert a chest tube in order to evacuate the blood from the patient's chest cavity and to reinflate her collapsed lungs. The nurses set up the instruments and equipment while the doctor began draping the patient with a sterile sheet. At that moment, the first of many units of packed red blood cells and fresh frozen plasma was being checked and, using a device called the rapid infuser, transfused as quickly as possible.

During the few moments of the chest tube insertion, because the patient was now under a sterile field and there wasn't much for me to do besides adjust a few medications and watch the monitor, I finally had an opportunity to look at the situation in front of me.

The patient was a mess and the room was a mess. Bloody linen, overflowing garbage cans, over a dozen IV lines infusing various drugs and blood products, the ventilator chirping alarm warnings—it was chaos. But this was purposeful, organized chaos. I knew from my ICU experience the reason for all of this chaos. This was a person, with a life, family, and friends, and I hoped our efforts would not be in vain.

"I got it," I heard the surgeon say and was quickly brought back to reality. I handed him the tubing for the chest tube drainage system and connected it to wall suction. Immediately a liter of frank, or bright red, blood drained into the canister. I paged for a portable chest x-ray so that I could confirm correct placement of the chest tube and continued to closely monitor her vital signs while the chest tube was being sutured in place. I drew repeated blood gases to ensure ventilation was optimal and discussed with the RT the appropriate adjustments to be made on the ventilator. The monitor was beginning to read near-normal signs of life: HR 110, BP 100/55, O_2 Sat at 98 percent. It looked like the situation was improving.

However, there was another worrisome sign: my patient was continuing to bleed from the wounds all over her body. I started changing her dressings, beginning at the open laceration to her left knee and lower leg, likely from the bumper of the car. I applied a silk gauze hemostat, which helps in clotting, directly to the wound in the hopes of easing some of the ongoing bleeding. I worked my way up her body, cleaning and dressing each skin tear and scrape. I rinsed her mouth, which was full of blood, and packed her bleeding nose. I applied small bandages to the cut above her brow and wiped more blood from her face. Despite her gruesome injuries, I could tell she was a pretty, well-groomed woman. She had manicured and polished nails; her long hair even now had some evident style.

I performed another neurological assessment. There were no improvements, no signs that she was waking up. Her pupils were equal and reactive to light, but her score on the Glasgow Coma Scale was a 3—the lowest possible score. She was not moving nor opening her eyes. She was completely unresponsive. The situation was looking very grim.

We still didn't know her identity. She was a nameless accident victim.

She began to shiver. I tried to take her temperature but it was so low it was undetectable. I called for an electric warming blanket and set it to high. The portable x-ray arrived and using full CTL (cervical, thoracic, and lumbar) spine precautions, four of us rolled the patient onto the board.

By this point, the patient's face had swollen extensively from her injuries as well as the fluids we had infused. It would have been difficult for anyone, even her family, to recognize her. Her eyelids were swollen and a deep red-purple. Her face had swollen around the ties holding her endotracheal tube in place. She had a large hematoma extending from her right shoulder down her chest and abdomen. As I did another visual head-to-toe assessment, I suddenly recognized the marking across her lower abdomen and pelvis. It was tire tracks. I was completely taken aback. The room fell silent, as though everyone around me noticed the same marking at the same time. A knot formed in my stomach. I wasn't ready to acknowledge that the car that hit this poor woman had in fact rolled over her. I didn't know what to think or how to react. I remember feeling angry but there wasn't time and I knew it wouldn't be appropriate to become emotional.

We had to get her off the x-ray board. I secured her head and cervical spine and on the count of three we rolled her. Suddenly, the patient began deteriorating again. She began to lose more blood than we could replace and her left pupil had now blown. It was fixed and dilated.

In less than four hours, I had gone from giggling with colleagues to caring for a patient with major traumatic injuries, and now, most certainly, to witnessing a tragic loss of life.

Still, I continued to do everything in my power to ensure that this patient would survive at least until her family arrived and had a chance to say good-bye. The doctor was aware I had increased her meds to nearly triple that of the recommended doses in order to try to maintain her vitals. I continued to give fluid boluses, alternating between saline and blood transfusions. She began to have arrhythmias despite my frequent checks and corrections of her serum electrolyte (sodium, potassium, calcium, magnesium, and phosphate) imbalances.

Finally, the call came. My patient's next of kin had been located. Our "Jane Doe" was Tracy Hammond. I braced myself as I went out to the hallway to meet her family. There was just one visitor, a man close in age to the patient, tall, with a noticeably strong build but looking weak with fear. I introduced myself and briefly described Tracy's injuries, trying to prepare him for what he would see when he entered the room: the ventilator, the monitor, tubes running in and out of his loved one's body, the bruising. As I spoke, his expression remained flat. He didn't say a word, only nodded yes when I asked if he was ready to come to the bedside.

I had done my best to make Tracy as presentable as possible, wiping off the blood, changing the oozing dressings, and covering her shocking wounds with pristine linen, but there was no denying it—it was a tragic scene and despite my efforts, she looked horrible.

The two nurses who I had left at the bedside to monitor and titrate drugs stopped and stepped away; now, the visitor took precedence. Peter, as I later learned, was Tracy's fiancé. They had recently moved to the city, leaving their families for job opportunities, so Peter was her only local next of kin. He approached the bed slowly and stood at a distance, staring at her.

I had the doctor paged and arranged for a conference room so that the three of us could discuss the situation. When the doctor arrived, I directed Peter to the room, discreetly grabbing a box of tissues on my way in. We sat down and Dr. Roberts introduced himself and offered his sympathy. He ran through, in lay terms, the full extent of Tracy's injuries and that they were likely too extensive for her to survive. He told Peter straight out that Tracy was going to die.

Peter sat there, with very little visible emotion, only rubbing his hands together as he listened. He was asked to decide whether we should continue a probably futile resuscitation or begin the process of withdrawal. Peter had very few questions but asked if he could have a minute to gather his thoughts. Dr. Roberts and I left the room and returned to Tracy Hammond's bedside. We stood at the foot of the bed in silence, waiting for instruction on how to proceed. In the meantime, despite our efforts, it looked like the decision would be made for us—Tracy was "declaring herself."

Not yet allowed to give up, we pressed on, increasing drips and hanging yet another fluid bolus, but it was becoming clear that Tracy was going to die. Peter stood in the doorway of Tracy's room. His eyes were red from crying. He said he had spoken with Tracy's parents and sister, who all lived in Montreal, and they all agreed. "Tracy wouldn't want to be this way," he said and asked for everything to be stopped, for us to now leave her alone. He walked over to her side and this time reached for her hand. Then he began tearing up; he kissed her forehead and walked out of the room.

Peter couldn't bear to stay for long. He was clearly uncomfortable being in the hospital and seeing Tracy in that state. I followed him out to the waiting room to make sure he was okay. He told me they had been engaged for two years but were so busy they still hadn't set a date. I tried to comfort him with all the clichés I could think of, but I don't think either of us bought it. He thanked me and, shaking my hand, said he couldn't stay and watch her die. That was it. He left; it was now up to me to be with Tracy in her dying moments.

The doctor was at my desk, writing orders in the chart and documenting the meeting with Peter. I walked back into the room and began turning off the drips. I grabbed a face cloth and again wiped the blood from Tracy's face. I had never met or spoken to her, yet I felt a definite personal connection. We were so close in age. I couldn't understand how Peter could leave, but I certainly wouldn't let Tracy be alone. I pulled a chair to the side of the bed, dropped the side rail down, and sat holding her hand. I watched the monitor display her changing heart rhythm; her blood pressure was dropping. It wasn't long before the various alarms began to ring. I stood up and checked her carotid. Tracy was dead.

I felt someone behind me holding my shoulders; it was Steve, one of the nurses who had been helping me. Neither of us said anything; we didn't need to. Together, we collected the equipment and washed her body before wrapping it. When I finished my charting, it was 4:30 A.M. and I was exhausted. The rest of the night was quiet. At 7:15 I changed out of uniform and left the hospital. I took an alleyway and barely made the corner off the main road before I broke down sobbing. I cried the whole way home.

Visiting Hours

~

Mary Malone-Ryan, RN, BN

IT WAS SUNDAY NIGHT. I drove to work, passing as usual the Catholic church that always looked so solemn beside the road, and did my ritual of blessing myself as I asked God if He could again do rounds with me this night shift. I also asked that He give me an extra dose of patience and wisdom tonight because I'd been unable to rest that afternoon before night shift. If I can get in a nap before work, it helps me work well during the night.

When I got to the ICU, I noticed that Room 286 was full of family members. This was unusual at shift change—to be honest, it was highly unusual in our ICU because the visiting hours were clearly defined and we went to great lengths to enforce this rule. Why are they here after visiting hours? I wondered to myself. I looked up at the assignment board and realized that that was my patient in Room 286.

I sat down, and the RN from the day shift who was about to give me her report broke away from the family to tell me, "Oh, Mary, I'm sorry to leave this with you, but we had to wait until all the family members were present." She pulled up a chair and sat beside me at the nursing station. We huddled together as she opened the patient's chart. The doctor's order answered my question regarding the family's presence after hours. "EXTUBATE this evening with all the family members present at patient's bedside," it read. That simple directive didn't come close to capturing what lay before me, my patient, and his family, in the long night ahead.

The day RN explained why she had not extubated her patient: "He's Hmong," she said. "They have a tradition of dressing a dying person in his own clothes before he dies, and they're not finished yet." I glanced at my watch; it was 6:48. This poor family doesn't even know me, I thought to myself. As far as they're concerned, I'm a complete stranger, and soon I'll be the one coming in to take their loved one off the ventilator. Soon after, he will die. I, the stranger, will be trying to offer them comfort during this tragic time in their lives.

Mr. Chu was 51 years old. He had a wife and six children. He had had a lung transplant a year ago and now a massive bleed in his head had caused so much damage that there was very little brain activity. The RN accompanied me to Room 286, hugged the wife, and introduced me to the family. "This is Mary. She will be your husband's nurse tonight."

I will also be *your* nurse tonight, I thought to myself. That's one thing I've learned in my long career as an ICU nurse: in these situations, the family is as much a part of your concern as the patient is.

Mr. Chu's small body was hooked up to the familiar intravenous pumps and monitors, as well as the ventilator. But he was dressed in unfamiliar garb: the green hospital gown was replaced with a gray suit and white shirt, and a beautiful brightly colored cloak was underneath him. His wife and his mother were meticulously making sure every button was buttoned and every zipper was zippered. The wife looked at me, "I cannot get his pants all the way on; could you help me?" I looked down: the Foley catheter was the obstacle. So, with every family member's eyes on me, I ever so gently manipulated the catheter through his pants, allowing them to zipper and button the pants. The wife then pulled the cloak up over his shoulders and nodded to her eldest son. The son said, "We are ready."

I began to perform my initial assessment. Pupils were dilated, no reaction to light; chest sounds were clear but decreased to the bases; heart sounds S_1 and S_2 were audible; no bowel sounds; no pulses detectable in the feet; there was trace edema and mottling at the tips of his toes.

Then it was time. The decision had been made: everyone was in agreement that to continue life support would have no benefit for Mr. Chu. It would only forestall his inevitable death. To continue with these futile measures would not, in this case, be the compassionate or dignified thing to do.

The first thing I had to do was pull out the endotracheal tube that was keeping oxygen flowing into his lungs. This wasn't like so many other times when I had extubated patients because they had been successfully weaned off the ventilator. This time there would be no success.

God, please guide me with my words and actions.

As I explained to the family what I was going to do, I slid my hand behind the ventilator and switched it off. A wave of silence fell across the room. I positioned myself at the head of the bed and extubated Mr. Chu. He started to make snoring sounds with each fast, shallow breath. The snoring sounded eerie to the family. In distress, they looked to me for explanation, reassurance. I felt unsettled too, because although I knew I had not caused this, I was the one that allowed it to happen. I offered to give my patient an analgesic that might decrease the snoring, but the family refused. I then offered a comparison to him snoring while asleep at home. This notion seemed to give them some peace.

Within moments after extubation, the cardiac monitor showed that Mr. Chu's heart rate was increasing to a sinus tachycardia of 148 beats per minute. I adjusted the alarm settings and repeated my assessment. There was no change. I tried patiently to answer the family's questions. But it was the question one of the younger sons put to me that was the most difficult to answer: "He is breathing on his own now and the monitor shows his heart is still working. Is it possible he could survive this?"

His words saddened me, because I knew he was looking for hope and I wasn't certain what I could offer. I had cared for many dying patients and their families before and I knew what I had to say and, most importantly, what to not say. I felt grateful at that moment for having my many years of experience to draw upon. "Your father has suffered a major bleed in his head. All of the tests—the MRIs, the CT scans, and the EEGs—have shown that there has been so much damage to his brain that he will not survive. His shallow breathing shows that his brain is not working to keep him alive. I am so sorry; but your father is dying with dignity. He is so blessed to have such a loving family."

I scanned the room. They all seemed to be processing what I'd just said. Without waiting for any more questions or comments, I excused myself to check on my other patient.

I returned to Room 286 frequently over the course of the night, bringing extra chairs, boxes of tissues, and cold drinks for the family. I continued to assess my patient's condition, jotting down vital signs and suction-ing from his mouth the oral secretions that he was unable to swallow.

For the family, the wait was on.

Seven hours passed; the family continued to hold their vigil. By 3 A.M., the physical and emotional exhaustion was visible on their faces. Suddenly, as I stood outside the door, charting the hourly vital signs, I heard screams from the room. I rushed in. Mr. Chu's breathing pattern had dramatically changed. He was gasping. It sounded like a struggle, but I knew it was the normal sound of the breaths of a dying person. His respirations were only about four or five a minute. I looked at the monitor. Mr. Chu's blood pressure was 54/36 and falling; the heart rhythm showed a wide, complex bradycardia. I rushed to the monitor to turn off all the alarms; they were no longer needed. All the family was looking at the monitor.

I knew my role. I had been here before.

I gently directed the family to focus on Mr. Chu and told them that the end was now very near. The family wailed, dropping their heads on his body; his wife franti-cally kissed his face, professing her love for him. I could feel a knot grow in my throat, tears forming in my eyes. I knew what was happening to me: I felt a measure of their sorrow. Twenty-two years as a nurse and it still happens to me. We nurses do our work, perform our important tasks, but we feel it, too.

I turned back to the monitor. Asystole. There were no more heartbeats. I discreetly turned off the monitor and, as the family watched, I auscultated his lungs and heart. There were no breath sounds, no heart sounds. "He is gone now," I told them. I hugged each family member in turn and allowed them to stay with their loved one's body as long as they wished.

The patient's and family's wishes had been carried out, and I had helped to make that happen. Very sad, but very satisfying to me, in my life as an ICU nurse: I could help make it possible for all the family members to be present at the patient's bedside in his last hours and moments, and to find some measure of peace.

Sick Kids

~

Linda L. Lindeke, PhD, RN, CNP

I WAS 23 YEARS OLD and had moved 3,000 miles to work at Toronto's The Hospital for Sick Children (Sick Kids'), the most famous children's hospital in the country. It was 1971. Wanting to challenge myself as much as I could, I asked to work in the ICU. This hospital was world renowned because it had pioneered some innovative procedures and was well-known as a world-class center for performing many experimental, cutting-edge open-heart surgeries for children. I remember hearing stories about the miracles performed for "blue babies" and about the surgical procedures that saved children's lives. When I was in third grade, I had known a little boy named Eddy, who was in my class and had to come to school in a wagon. He died that year. Eddy could have benefited from the particular kind of open-heart surgery that was only done at that time at Sick Kids' Hospital. It was from these experiences that I developed an interest in children's heart surgery from a very early age.

It was amazing to work in that hospital's ICU. Children arrived at the hospital from many continents. We cared for many patients from very wealthy families in the impoverished but oil-rich countries of Central and South America. We also cared for native children from the reserves of northern Canada whose parents were not able to fly down to be with them and thus, we, the nurses, became their proxy families. Daily I would look up from the bedside of a sick child and see a group of visiting doctors and nurses from other parts of the world who were touring our unit and learning about the care we gave and the techniques we used.

My experience working at this hospital, decades ago, has shaped my life and career. Teamwork is one of the most powerful lessons I learned. Children died daily in the ICU because the children who were the most severely ill were the ones who were transferred to this facility from near and far. We dealt with incredibly intense and heartbreaking situations, and because of the flat structure (meaning, there was little hierarchy; we all worked closely together) of the professional and support staff—our teamwork—we also saved countless lives. Staff turnover was low because we supported one another and gained tremendous satisfaction from caring for the children and families in the best possible way.

We were all on a first-name basis in the unit. Staff nurses were valued and their skills and responsibilities appreciated. The custodial staff was known by name and often formed relationships with the children and families, some of whom remained on our unit for months. Teamwork was wordless at times, and very verbally expressed at other times. Of the many powerful situations I remember, here is one I still learn from.

As I gained nursing skills, both intellectual and manual, the level of complexity of my daily assignments gradually increased. I had to know when a subtle change in a child's breathing indicated a post-surgical complication of pneumonia or internal bleeding. I had to be able to manage ventilators, tubes, lines, medications, and various procedures unthinkingly, automatically, so that I could be simultaneously comforting the child and communicating with the family during the daily care.

As the level of my responsibilities advanced, I was under the close supervision of experienced nurses. After a while, they deemed me ready to be the nurse who cared for a child directly out of the operating room after open-heart surgery. Children did not go to a recovery room after surgery because our ICU was equipped to care for them in the post-anesthetic phase; that way they would not need to be moved a second time. The sickest children and those undergoing the most complex surgeries were the first on the daily operating room schedule. The ICU routine for post-op care was that the assigned nurse spent the time prior to the patient's return from surgery setting up the room and doing as many things in advance as possible, so that she or he could immediately care for the patient returning from the OR. That meant preparing all the medications, intravenous solutions, bandages, charting forms, and other equipment. I had done all those things many times in my supervised orientation and knew the drill. I was ready. Because I was ready ahead of time, I spent my spare time relieving other nurses as they went on breaks and helping nurses who needed an extra hand with their patients.

Then the call came that my patient was coming out of the OR. The bed was wheeled into the room. The child's small body was barely visible beneath the tubes, machines, and dressings of the entire chest. My heart was racing and my adrenaline surging as I put my training into practice, providing immediate care for this child and family during the critical post-operative phase. I was moving at top speed and thinking as fast as I could to be sure I was doing everything in the right order and with correct procedure.

Suddenly I looked up and saw Marion, the calmest and most understated nurse I believe I have ever met. She gave a small smile and went to the other side of the child's bed. Without a word she reached over and took off the blood pressure cuff that I had just put on the little arm. Carefully and slowly she repositioned and connected the cuff to the wall-mounted equipment. She then gave me a penetrating glance and a small smile, and walked away.

What was Marion doing at that moment? Why can I re-create that scene in crystal-clear detail? Because in my rush to remember all the tasks I needed to do to give this small, sick child the best care I could provide, I failed to pay attention to detail. Marion slowed me down; I had to look at my own behavior. In fact, in this high-stress situation, I wasn't being effective overall. A reading from a misapplied blood pressure cuff is worse than no reading at all. Blood pressure is a key indicator of post-operative bleeding, septic shock, and other serious complications. One of the first things I had learned in nursing school was how to take a blood pressure reading, and now, at a time of critical importance, I had made a mistake in a simple task, and that mistake could have jeopardized my patient.

I learned from Marion that being a mentor and role model is subtle work, and profoundly significant work: powerful mentoring can occur in a brief moment, if the mentor is a wise and internally grounded, caring person. Marion was head nurse for a reason. She possessed qualities that were not apparent on first meeting. She was not outgoing or flashy in her communication. She didn't take center stage and demonstrate her deep understanding of pathophysiology, quality improvement, or the latest administrative process, though she had all those areas of expertise. She knew how to be in the moment and how to connect to a person's inner core.

I continued to work in the ICU for a year and a half and have countless other moments of deep learning that stay with me to this day. I left to become a nursing educator when an enticing opportunity came my way. I still tend to rush when I'm in a new or stressful situation; I tend to respond too quickly, in ways that are less precise or thoughtful than if I had been more deliberate in my actions. I continue to struggle with that tendency and tell myself to slow down and make sure that small but essential details are attended to.

There are many, many more stories that I could write about this ICU era of my life. Perhaps I will write more. But the story of Marion's wisdom and mentoring needs to be told. Thank you, Marion.

Ray Can't Get No Satisfaction

~

Lisa Huntington, RN

A<small>FTER OVERDOSING</small> on crack cocaine and alcohol at a Rolling Stones concert, Ray, a 42-year-old unemployed truck driver, ended up in our ICU to dry out overnight. He was unconscious, barely responsive to deep pain stimulus, and not breathing at all, so we had to fully ventilate him. As he began to wake up, he got restless and needed close monitoring. He kept making yanking motions to indicate that he wanted the breathing tube out, but he wasn't awake enough or breathing on his own enough to have the uncomfortable apparatus removed yet. As with most overdose patients he began to wake up in fits and starts, at times thrashing around on the bed. We couldn't sedate him because we wanted him to wake up so that we could extubate him, yet we were all at risk of him causing injury to us caring for him with one of his kicks or jabs, so we had to put him in four-point restraints: both arms and both legs had to be tied down.

Ray finally woke up and, like Hospital Houdini, managed to slip his right hand out of its restraint. The first thing he did was pull out his breathing tube, setting off various bedside alarms. My partner for the day, Shilpa, a very petite middle-aged Pakistani nurse, got to him first, but she was no match for his 220 pounds of drunken fury. She tried to calm him down, suction his lungs, and assess his breathing. He had a strong cough and was able to get out a few words (swearing and threats, mostly). "Listen, lady, I gotta record as long as my arm, so call the cops if you wanna!" He then promptly passed out.

"I think I will let sleeping dogs remain lying down, so to speak," Shilpa said. She enjoyed trying out various English idioms and using them in her own way.

I tried to settle Ray and managed to convince him that if he'd sit up, do the deep breathing and coughing exercises I had instructed him in, using an incentive spirometer device designed to inflate his lungs, and go along with other chest physio exercises, we might be able to spare him an unpleasant re-intubation. In his semi-stuporous, semi-lucid state, he managed to convince me that he'd cooperate. By then, it was time for my lunch break and the ICU finally seemed quiet enough for me to take it. Shilpa would be able to manage on her own, I figured.

I had no sooner walked down the hallway, away from the ICU, when I heard Shilpa cry out, "Lisa-girl! Come back! Help me! All of hell is breaking loose!"

I ran back to find Shilpa cowering in the corner. Ray had managed to spring loose from all four of his restraints. He'd jumped out of bed and ripped out his IV. Blood was dripping all over the bed and the floor. Even worse, he had ripped out his arterial line and bright red blood was gushing out of his radial artery. He'd even pulled out his Foley catheter; there was blood dripping from his penis due to that rough method of removal. Ouch, I thought, wincing at the sight. There he stood beside the bed, naked now, having torn off his hospital gown, ECG electrodes hanging from his chest but disconnected from the monitor, teetering on one leg, the other still tethered to the footboard. He was still confused but had cleverly managed to grab a pair of suture scissors and was madly trying to cut the last flannel restraint binding his foot.

I tried reasoning with Ray, but he was just getting more agitated. I had no choice but to call a Code White over the public announcement system. The security squad would help with our violent patient. I managed to get close enough to Ray so that I could clamp some pressure on that bleeding artery, while Shilpa tried to cover up Ray's private parts, but he didn't care about that and waved her away.

"I just want to get the fuck outta here!"

Two security guards finally turned up with the nursing supervisor. They donned disposable gloves, crossed their arms, and stood just outside the door, looking bored. They couldn't do much more than we were doing.

We all tried negotiating with Ray, trying to calm him down and make him behave, to no avail. He was staggering around, mumbling and getting wobbly on his feet. Finally, he dropped the scissors and fell back onto his bed. I untied the last restraint and covered him back up. Shilpa promised him that he could have a drink as soon as she checked his blood pressure and oxygen level and put a bandage where his IV had been and a pressure dressing over his arterial line site.

Ray no longer needed to be in the ICU. He certainly needed something; I wasn't sure what, but it wasn't the ICU. The guards said we could call them back if we needed them. I was about to find the resident to write transfer orders and have Ray sent to a medical floor. But Ray would have none of that. He wanted to go home.

"I want out of here, now! Where're my clothes?" He was getting restless again and there was no reasoning with him. The decision was made that he could be safely discharged home if a responsible adult came to pick him up. We managed to track down a brother who lived about

an hour away who said he'd come around to pick up Ray
. . . eventually. Until then, Ray remained in our care. He
scowled at that. "Well, if I have to stay here, I'm gonna
need a drink," he mumbled.

Shilpa, always helpful, brought him a paper cup of
apple juice.

"Not the drink I had in mind," Ray said.

"You can lead horse to juice but cannot force him to
take the drink," she said, with a giggle.

Ray drank the juice, then immediately announced,
"I need to take a piss." I offered him a urinal, explaining
that he was still too shaky to walk to the bathroom. I
just hoped he wouldn't throw it. Shilpa grabbed the full
bottle just before Ray passed out again on the bed. "The
cup is running over," she said, and we both tried to hold
back our laughter, but no matter, as Ray had dozed off
to sleep.

Suddenly, he woke up with a start. "Where are my
pants?" I gingerly handed the booze-stained, cigarette
smoke–infused garment to him. As he shakily pulled on
the pants, about ten dollars in change and three guitar
picks fell out onto the floor. I helped him get dressed and
then brought him a sandwich.

"Thanks, ma'am," he whispered.

An hour before the end of my shift, Dave, Ray's
brother, finally arrived. Unfortunately, he seemed even
drunker than Ray. I prayed he wasn't driving. It was

unusual to discharge a patient from the ICU directly home. Most of our patients go to a step-down unit and then to the floor before going home, but Ray had gone from a critical condition to his normal, sober but chronic, alcoholic state in less than 24 hours and was ready to resume his "normal" life straight from the ICU.

As Ray walked out of the ICU door and made his way to the elevator with his brother, I couldn't resist asking him the question that had been on my mind.

"How were the Rolling Stones?"

Ray turned back to me with a big, semi-toothless grin, gave me a thumbs-up, and rasped out a classic, Canadian-style answer, "They were fuckin' *eh*!"

Almost

≈

Bella Medeiros Manos, RN

WHEN I FIRST STARTED in the ICU I was terrified. I always worried: What will the next shift bring? Will I be able to handle what's thrown at me? Do I have the right stuff to be an ICU nurse? Before the start of each shift, there would be a tight knot in my stomach that just wouldn't go away. I would walk into the ICU, glance at the assignment board posted near the nursing station, read the name of the patient listed beside my name, and think, This is the name of the person whose life will be entrusted into my care for the next 12 hours. I would walk slowly to my patient's room. "It's good to feel fear," the older nurses would say so confidently. "That's the way you should feel when you start out in the ICU.

"It builds character," they would tell me, as they went about their work.

It was easy for them to say that. They had years of experience under their belts, just like I do now. Nurses can be harsh with their young. For a long time, I always felt I had to prove myself to them. But the real reason I felt such fear working in the ICU was that despite all my new ICU skills, acquired in a six-week crash course on critical care, along with my new knowledge base and repertoire of advanced skills such as mechanical ventilation and CVVHD (a form of hemodialysis), hemodynamic monitoring (which involves pulmonary artery catheters, cardiac outputs, titrating inotropes, and cardiac rhythm interpretation), I grasped pretty quickly how enormous are the responsibilities of the ICU. Patients' lives are literally in our hands.

Another challenge of the ICU has to do with working as part of the larger multidisciplinary team. In the ICU, nurses are expected to present our findings and recommendations about our patients to everyone on rounds. "Everyone" includes staff doctors; residents from specialists such as anesthesiology, general surgery, or cardiology, pharmacists; social workers; respiratory therapists; dietitians; physiotherapists; and others. It was new for me to communicate my nursing knowledge with all of those other professionals. I prayed to not sound like a babbling fool when my turn came to present my patient! In those early days, when everything was so daunting and scary, I kept thinking, What have I got myself into? Couldn't I have chosen an easier path?

I have cared for many patients in my twenty years of ICU practice. Not every patient grabs you and leaves you with a lasting impression, but some do. There is one patient I will never forget. I was on a night shift and still very new to critical care. I can still feel a flicker of the fear I felt as I entered her room and still recall a particular stale, sour odor and the feeling that I wanted to run and never come back.

I was assigned to care for Sabrina Sanchez, a young woman with breast cancer. When I looked at her chart, I saw she was exactly the same age as I was—24. When I saw her colorful head scarf of yellow and green daisies, I knew it was to cover her bald head. She'd lost her hair from chemotherapy. I saw how pale she was and checked her lab results. Sure enough, her hemoglobin was very low. I wondered if I would be giving her a blood transfusion that night. She was very thin, with deep-sunk eyes and no eyelashes. Her lashes had fallen out, too, like the rest of her hair, from the chemotherapy. Her exposed eyes, bony frame, and pale skin made her look so vulnerable. I didn't know if I was up to the challenge of caring for someone who looked so sad and needy. A part of me wanted to run away. My first thought was to ask for a different patient assignment. The prospect of caring for this patient felt emotionally overwhelming. But the day nurse had already started giving her handover report to me and I felt I couldn't interrupt her. Besides, I didn't want to show my fear. There was no way out. To cope, I focused on her disease.

Sabrina's cancer must be very aggressive, I reasoned, because although she had been recently diagnosed, she already had metastases to her brain and bones. She was in the icu because of sepsis—overwhelming infection—and pneumonia, too, both of which she'd gotten because of the immunosuppressive effects of the chemotherapy. She was on a ventilator and needed close monitoring, aggressive fluid replacement, and iv antibiotics.

At the end of her report, the day nurse told me a very important piece of information. That very day, Sabrina, our patient, had made a decision. She had requested that all treatment be stopped. She wanted to be allowed to die. Because it was a big decision, and one that couldn't be rushed, nothing was going to be done that night. My job was to keep everything going until the morning. If Sabrina still felt the same way the next day, everything would be stopped and treatment would be withdrawn.

Thoughts came rushing at me as I listened to the day nurse tell me this information. I looked at our patient. Why are you giving up? I wanted to say. You can't do this. Don't make this choice. I looked at the day nurse, who was still giving me her report, but I could barely listen because thoughts were swirling in my head: She can't make this choice! She's my age exactly. She must be depressed and not thinking right. She's in no state of mind to make this fateful decision. We can't give up on her, even if she wants to give up on herself. Someone stop this! This is a mistake. Have you all lost your minds?

But I kept my thoughts to myself. I couldn't say those things out loud. I couldn't tell anyone how upset I felt over her decision. I had to find a way to deal with my feelings. I was the one with the problem.

I began that shift as I began every shift, with a methodical head-to-toe assessment of my patient. I took refuge in my critical thinking skills and rational, logical mind. They helped me to stay focused and keep my emotions in check, but my private thoughts kept intruding: We're the same age. I'm healthy and happy. Today, while I've been planning my upcoming wedding, you've been spending the day planning your good-bye to your family and friends.

I felt overcome with sadness and despair at this woman's situation and her decision. I'd wanted to be an ICU nurse to help people and make things better. I wanted to save lives. What this young woman was doing made no sense to me. I could barely look her in the eye as I took care of her.

I stayed focused on her body. I saw how the endotracheal tube was cutting into her dry, cracked lips. I saw how the skin on her left breast was still burned from recent radiation therapy. Her abdomen was concave from not being able to eat any of the foods she probably, just like me, enjoyed—ice cream, good greasy fries, café latte loaded with whipped cream. Sabrina no longer wanted these things. She only wanted her suffering to stop. I was about to ask her why, but stopped myself. I suppose I could figure out the answer, but I could not accept it. I guess I didn't ask her because I didn't want to hear her say it. She wasn't able to speak because she was intubated, but I didn't hand her a clipboard and ask her to write me a note, because I didn't want to face what she might write there.

As the night wore on, I continued to do my best to hide my feelings. I gave Sabrina her medications and took hourly vital signs. I made adjustments on the ventilator. I even took blood work and sent it off to the laboratory. I washed my patient's hair and glossed her lips. I went about doing everything I could to keep my patient pain free, comfortable, warm, washed, and well groomed. I cared for her as if she were a patient who we had every reason to believe was going to get better.

All the while, I kept thinking, How do you plan that today will be "that day"? What if she changes her mind? Can I help her change her mind? Maybe I could help her choose to live. I counted the minutes until the end of my shift.

As morning approached, I began my end-of-shift routines: tallying fluid balances, emptying drains, tidying the room, and doing last-minute turns and comfort measures. As I worked, Sabrina woke fully. She began to bite on her breathing tube as if to cut off her oxygen supply. Each time she did that, her airway was occluded, the alarm on the ventilator went off, and I silenced it. I begged her to stop, but she was determined. I tried to force her jaw to stay open. I attempted to insert a plastic oral airway but was unsuccessful. I was about to give her some light sedation to make her stop fighting the ventilator, but she shook her head furiously when I suggested that. Is this how she'll go? I thought. I can't let this happen! I can't have someone die right in front of me by her own hand when I'm the nurse on duty! Sabrina continued to struggle against the ventilator, clamping off the tube in her mouth with her teeth so that no air could enter her lungs. She pulled at the tube, trying to rip it out of her lungs. In panic, I pulled the call bell and screamed for help.

Sabrina was starting to turn blue from lack of oxygen. Her mouth was clamped down so tight that no air was getting into her lungs. The ventilator alarm kept going off. I knew what she was doing. She was determined to die, ready to go then and there, in this brutal way, right before my eyes. Again I tried to pry her teeth apart, but they were clenched down on the tube. Her actions were louder than any words. She was furious at me for trying to stop her. She grabbed the scarf from her head and threw it across the room. I held on tight to keep the endotracheal tube in place so that she would continue to receive oxygen. I held down her arms to prevent her from violently pulling out the endotracheal tube and damaging her airway and vocal cords. Soon, others came to help and we managed to keep the tube in place. I was shaking by the time everyone arrived.

When my shift ended, an hour or so later, I left Sabrina looking out the window, her bald head exposed. Tears were running down her face. It was a beautiful spring morning. Trees outside her room were in full bloom. A new day was beginning for me, but this young woman's life was about to end. . . . *Today will be her last day.* There was nothing I could do but accept her decision.

As I gave my report to the day nurse coming on, I knew I had failed this patient. I was there to support patients in their choices, even if their choices were not the ones I would make. I walked out of the hospital that day a different person, a different nurse. And to this very day I remember Sabrina Sanchez. I wasn't there for her death—the other nurses told me it occurred later that day—but almost.

Three A.M.

~

Sarah Burns, RN, BSCN

THE STRETCHER WITH THE CARDIAC MONITOR was parked outside Mr. McGovern's room. The bottom shelf of the stretcher was full, packed with IV tubing, bags of fluid, a portable blood pressure cuff, and all the emergency drugs. We call this stretcher the Cadillac.

"Going on a road trip?" I asked Alice. She was standing near the sink in Mr. McGovern's room, mixing water with all the pills she'd crushed.

She looked over at Mr. McGovern and rolled her eyes. He lay there, mounds of pinky white flesh, arms sprawled out, filling the bed. "We're going to head CT," Alice said.

I looked down at the flow sheet. He weighed 359 pounds. "What's the weight limit?" I mouthed.

"I guess the table can hold this much if he's spread out," Alice whispered. "Like if he were five foot two, they couldn't do it."

"When are you going?" I asked.

She looked up at the clock. "They want us down there in fifteen minutes."

"Want me to page respiratory?"

"Rochelle's on," Alice said. "She's going to finish her treatments and she'll be over. Could you call CT though, and tell them to send *two* transport people? Look at all this junk." She waved her hand toward the six IV pumps, the ventilator, all the tubes and wires.

I called CT, checked on Mr. Livingston, and returned to the room. Alice had the Cadillac lined up next to the bed, the IV pumps wheeled up to the head of the bed, out of the way. Drew was disconnecting the cables from the monitor, turning stopcocks, flushing lines.

"Maybe you should just take him in the bed," I suggested. "That way you'll only have to move him twice."

Alice looked at the Cadillac, then at Mr. McGovern. "Yeah, if we have two transporters—yeah, that's a better idea."

I hooked Mr. McGovern up to the portable monitor and lifted it off the Cadillac.

"Just moving your leg over a little," Drew said. He pushed the right leg over as far as he could and I set the monitor down on the bed. Alice put the box of emergency drugs by the left leg and we stuck the blood pressure cuff and the chart up near Mr. McGovern's shoulders. Then Rochelle walked in with a new oxygen tank and an ambu bag. Drew wedged the oxygen tank between the side rail and the monitor. I took down the pressure bags and laid them on Mr. McGovern's arms.

Now the bed was full. Rochelle had disconnected him from the ventilator and was bagging him with the ambu bag, but still no transport people.

"I can go down with you," I said to Alice.

We hoisted the pumps up and hung them on the side rails, but that made the bed too wide and we kept bumping into things. One pump had a continuous blood pressure infusion, one was an antiarrhythmic, two were infusing antibiotics, another had a sedative, and the sixth line was the med-line, which I mentally took special note of: I knew it would be the line I'd use to push drugs in case of an emergency. So Alice hung three of the pumps from the headboard and I pushed the other three. Rochelle kept bagging and I steered the bed. We made it to the elevator but we had to take the pumps off the bed so the elevator doors could shut. Rochelle was squeezed in at the head of the bed, bagging Mr. McGovern; Alice was at the foot, watching the monitor and the pumps. "I'll take the stairs," I told them.

When we got downstairs we pulled the bed and all the equipment out of the elevator. I'm always afraid the wheel of the bed will fall into the gap between the hospital floor and the elevator doors. The space is exactly the width of the bed wheel. I'm good at imagining disasters. When I'm snow skiing, I imagine hitting one of those moguls and falling smack on my back, rupturing my kidney, bleeding internally. Water skiing is worse: I think the rope will accidentally get wrapped around my wrist and the boat will drag me that way. I know I'll have to curb these paranoid thoughts if I ever have a child.

We traveled up and down the halls twice before we found the right CT room. Mr. McGovern was doing fine, his chest rising and falling with the breaths Rochelle gave him. I took over bagging while Rochelle ran back upstairs to get the ventilator.

The CT technician emerged from the other room. He was pale, dressed in a white uniform, sort of like a pant suit. His hair was sandy colored and his glasses were too big for his face. "How much does this gentleman weigh?" he asked.

"Three fifty-nine," Alice said

"Pounds?"

"Yes, pounds."

"Well, I don't know why they even send these patients down here. Our weight limit is three hundred and twenty pounds."

Alice quickly brought him up to speed on the height times weight, square mass of flesh rule and we moved him over to the CT table. He was heavy but at least he wasn't fighting us. I hate bringing people down who are moving all over the place, trying to sit up. Usually the doctors don't want to give them any sedatives because they don't want to "cloud" the mental status. That makes sense, but then you have these CT technicians telling you they can't do the study if the guy won't hold still. So you're caught in the middle, trying to please all parties and get the test done. It must be what middle management is like.

Alice found some Velcro straps in the cupboard and we swaddled Mr. McGovern's IV tubing and his arms up against his body. One pump started to beep and I pulled the Velcro strap off, straightened the IV line, and wrapped the arm back up; then another pump beeped. The technician crossed his arms and sighed.

"The battery is low on this one," Alice said. "Where can I plug it in?" She started toward the wall with the cord.

"Not there," he said, still with his arms across his chest. "The scanner needs to move back and you'll knock that pump right over."

"This is a level one trauma center!" I wanted to yell at him. "Lots of people are going to come down here with lots of machines to plug in. You need to have a PLAN!"

"Can I use this?" Alice pulled a power strip with a long cord from the corner. I admired her persistence and unflappable style.

"That's fine." He opened the door and went into the adjoining room to start the scanner.

"What a worm," Alice said. She handed me a pink lead apron and a little cellophane package.

"What's this?" I asked.

"Fruit roll-up." She wrapped the blue lead apron around herself and opened her own fruit roll-up. We leaned against the counter, three o'clock in the morning, eating our fruit roll-ups and watching Mr. McGovern get fed into the scanner. "What was everyone so worried about?" Alice laughed. "There's at least two millimeters to spare."

"Yeah, and we didn't even have to grease his sides to get him in." I popped the last of my fruit roll-up in my mouth and washed my hands.

"When did he come in?" I asked Alice.

"Three thirty. A neighbor found him in his apartment. But no drugs, no alcohol." Alice always grilled the ambulance drivers for details. "Bobby said he had stacks of newspapers and magazines everywhere in his apartment, like a path. It was hard to get the stretcher out. "

The worm pushed the door open. "We're finished," he reported.

"Did you see anything?" Alice asked him.

"I'm not at liberty to say." *Why was I not surprised?* I turned away from him and rolled my eyes at Alice. Then a transporter arrived and we pulled Mr. McGovern back over to his bed.

Same thing on the way up: Rochelle bagging, Alice watching the monitor and the lines, the transporter and I pushing the bed and the pumps. I sealed them all in the elevator and I took the stairs.

By the time I climbed the last set of steps, I was pretty winded. I walked through the door and right into complete chaos. The bed was halfway out of the elevator, the elevator alarming: Alice was kneeling on the bed doing chest compressions, Rochelle was bagging and the transporter was using the elevator phone.

"I'd like to report a Code Blue coming to seven east," the transporter said in a calm voice. "Yes sir," he said. "We're almost there." He hung up the phone and turned to Alice. "I know CPR, can I help?" he asked, just like in the CPR class—good for him. "We're good," Alice said. "But thanks," she smiled.

I helped the transporter extract the bed and the six IV pumps from the elevator. "You are a magnet for drama." I told Alice.

"You can't leave me alone for a second." She continued compressions. Her face was flushed, her blond ponytail swinging forward with each compression.

We rounded the corner and Drew was holding the door open; the doctors and the code team were coming through the door.

Our resident Jeremy arrived in wrinkled scrubs, running his hands through his hair. "What's this guy's story?"

"Sixty-seven years old," Alice said. She nodded to the transporter and he took over compressions. "Found down at home." I handed the CPR board in and opened a box of epinephrine. "History of coronary artery disease, had a bypass in '90, bilateral carotid endarterectomies." Alice climbed off the bed and on the count of three we all rolled Mr. McGovern onto the CPR board.

"Stop CPR," Jeremy said, stepping forward and feeling for a pulse. "Okay, let's keep going. And let's push some epi."

Alice pushed the epinephrine into the IV line I'd designated earlier as the "med-line" in which to push emergency drugs and opened the roller clamp to flush it in. The transporter continued compressions. He was tall and his technique looked smooth and effortless, like he was using one of those hand pumps for a camping mattress.

"We just went to head CT," Alice said. "His heart rate went up into the one-seventies for about a minute and then he dropped into the twenties, so we started CPR."

"Do you have a strip?" Jeremy asked

A EKG strip? We were in the elevator on a portable monitor. The transporter had called the arrest on the elevator phone. No, we didn't have a strip! "No," Alice answered calmly, and she grabbed another box of epinephrine. I guess I shouldn't be so hard on people; these interns get beeped out of a sound sleep and we expect them to think clearly and bound into action. We continued CPR, no pulse, more epinephrine, listened to the breath sounds, listened again, considered a cardiac tap. Finally Jeremy called it. At that moment, I had to leave to answer another patient's cd bell.

"Hi, Sam." He squeezed my hand.

"How are you?" I asked and he gave me the thumbs-up.

"Drew's busy," I told him. "But I can help you. Do you need suctioning?" He nodded. I hooked the ambu bag up to his trache but he reached up and squeezed the bag himself.

"Hey, pretty good," I said. He still had an arterial line in his right wrist, so he steadied the bag with that hand and pushed with the left. I suctioned him and hooked him back up to the ventilator. I spooned a few ice chips into his mouth, flipped his pillow, and turned off the light.

When I returned to Mr. McGovern's room, the code cart and the ventilator were gone. The drips had all been taken down and the pumps delivered to the dirty utility room. Alice was sitting on a chair next to the bed, the chart on her lap.

"Are they going to do an autopsy?" I asked.

"I think so. No one can get hold of the family, though." She picked up the chart, looked over the note, then signed her name.

I never know what to write for death notes; I usually just write what happened, what time the doctor pronounced the death, and whatever happened with the family or the patient belongings. One doctor I knew always wrote, "May he rest in peace," at the end of his note. I tried it once but it seemed awkward. Even though I felt it, it seemed preachy.

"His CT was a mess," Alice said.

"What?"

"Yeah, Jeremy just got the results. He had a huge stroke." Alice pulled her ponytail forward and ran her hand along it. "So I'm not sure what to do. I guess I'll just leave all the tubes in, in case they do an autopsy, and get him all cleaned up. I'll have to pin two sheets together—we'll never be able to wrap him in just one."

Alice went to get washcloths and I filled the basin with water. Since Mr. McGovern had just come in he didn't have any belongings in the cupboard, no cards on the wall, no pictures. I looked down at him, so big and pale. I wondered what he was thinking about right before his stroke. Maybe he was trying to read one of his newspapers. Funny that a lifetime of thoughts and memories can be cut off in a moment by a single clot of blood.

We cleaned up the body and I left the room to answer the phone. Alice followed me out and spread the sheets on an empty bed next door. I watched her bend at the waist, folding the edges of the sheets, pinning them together. Then with her thumb and forefinger she caught the top of her ponytail, and with a flick of her wrist, all her hair flew up and spread across her back. She balanced on her white clogs, folding, pinning, folding. Then, in one movement, she picked up the double sheet and twirled around.

I hung up the phone. "All set?" I asked her. And we went in to wrap Mr. McGovern and prepare his body to send to the morgue.

O, Holy Night!

~

Bob Hicks, RN, BSCN, BHSC

IT'S 11:57 P.M., Christmas Eve, and I'm at work in the ICU. As I get ready to perform another set of hourly vital signs on my patient, I glance out the window and see that a small snow flurry has started. There's something comforting about working in the hospital during the holiday season. Maybe it's the break from the hustle and bustle of the malls and of trying to squeeze in every last minute with family and friends, or maybe it is just the comfort of knowing that at the end of my long shift I'll have a nice warm bed at home waiting for me to crawl into.

My patient tonight is an elderly woman, almost 90 years old. I read in her chart that she happens to be a nun. She's devoted her entire life to the work of God, and now I am here to watch over her life and ensure her comfort while she's under my watch. It's my lucky night. What could be better than caring for a nun on Christmas? She is someone who, I imagine, spent a lifetime of work to guarantee her entrance into heaven. I'll have to ask her to remember to throw in a good word for me, I think to myself.

My patient, Bernice, was brought to the ICU after being found unconscious on the floor of her home. It was uncertain how long she had been lying there: possibly four or five days. Half of her body was covered in blackened, necrotic ulcers. She must have fallen, because she had completely fractured both her hip and her clavicle. There was also a small fracture in her skull, and she had a small cerebral bleed from which she is starting to recover. Now, finally, she is beginning to regain consciousness.

Bernice's vital signs are stable: heart rate 82, blood pressure 134/65, and temperature normal. She's in normal sinus rhythm with oxygen saturation 97 percent. She'd been extubated a few days earlier and is now on four liters of oxygen by nasal prongs. She is starting to wake up, but her mental status alternates between stuperous and confused. She moves her arms slightly and is unable to move her legs, possibly because they have become edematous—swollen to more than twice their size. She opens her eyes from time to time and stares blankly into space. Despite all of this, Bernice looks peaceful lying there in bed. She's in no obvious discomfort. In fact, for her, this state of hovering between life and death is probably closer to God than she's ever been, even though she's devoted a lifetime to the church.

I listen to her chest with my stethoscope and hear that it is starting to sound a lot worse than before. It is even worse than it was an hour ago, when I performed my initial shift assessment. When I try to clear away secretions, by suctioning her through her nose and at the back of her throat, I note that she has very weak gag and cough reflexes. Bernice is not nearly strong enough to protect her airway from these thick secretions. Her chest is noisy and I can hear coarse, scattered crackles throughout the lower half of her lung fields. I'm going to have to resort to more invasive measures to clear the secretions from her chest and upper airways. I absolutely hate doing this to my patients, especially ones like Bernice, who have been lucky enough to have lived 90 years and whose time to go peacefully will soon arrive. It's invasive and undignified, but it has to be done. She can't get proper oxygen exchange with all the thick fluid in the way, and she can't cough it out by herself. If I don't do this unpleasant procedure, she will likely have to be reintubated and put back onto mechanical ventilation, both of which will increase her risk of getting pneumonia. I know I have to do it.

When I was a novice nurse, new to the ICU, Karen, who was one of my preceptors and one of the strongest nurses I've known to date, taught me this technique. I've always looked up to her and modeled my nursing practice after hers. She always remained calm, always seemed to have an answer when dealing with the most difficult of situations, and, if she didn't, she knew exactly where to find the solution.

I take the Yankauer suction catheter (a rigid plastic oral suctioning device, approximately one foot long) and begin to clear the secretions from Bernice's mouth. I slowly inch the catheter toward the back of her throat to try to stimulate her weak gag reflex and get her to cough up the deep secretions from the bases of her lungs. *No luck.* Now onto the part I am reluctant to do. It is unpleasant, but I do it because I know the alternative, mechanical ventilation, carries worse risks than this brief, temporary discomfort.

At the back of Bernice's throat, I continue onward with the suction catheter; still nothing. She doesn't have the strength or alertness to cough. *She needs to cough.* I always try to think about how uncomfortable and invasive it must feel, but I don't really think anyone can properly imagine how it feels, no matter how hard they try. I push on farther down her throat. Still no reflex. I now have my hand just about all the way into her mouth and this rigid piece of plastic must be at least six inches down her throat; then I finally hit the spot. Bernice begins to gag slightly; then she is frantically coughing, trying to clear this foreign probe from her trachea. Halfway through the coughing fit her eyes open up, and now they are focused, as they had not been (until now) during her stay in the ICU. She looks squarely at me with a menacing glare.

"You son of a bitch!"

It was as though Bernice had been following the white light and, as she reached the end of her ascent, Saint Peter himself slammed the gates shut right in her face.

There are more secretions to be cleared. I move the catheter back into her mouth and start the process again.

"You son of a bitch," she snarls at me again, with a mixture of disgust and anger. The devout nun, now appearing to be possessed by Satan himself! She's ready to take me along with her to the afterlife, through the firing brigade of hell, to be seated in unrest at her right side for eternity! And then, after working so hard at clearing her chest, Bernice falls asleep.

Get some rest, Saint Bernice, I think to myself with a chuckle. I'll be with you for the rest of this night, caring for you and helping you to clear out your chest again in a few minutes. There's no rest for the weary ICU nurse.

In the morning, when my shift is over, I make my way back home, offering a Merry Christmas to Bernice, my fellow workers, to those who celebrate Christmas, and to those who don't.

Power and Voice

~

Sharon Reynolds, RN, BSCN, MHSC (bioethics)

My patient had been in the hospital many months, in and out of the ICU. We knew he was not going to get better and go home. I think, deep down, he knew this too. When I met him, his affect was flat. There was no animation in his face. When I asked him if he was comfortable I had to stand back a bit to watch for the very slight nod of his head, which one could easily miss if one wasn't watching closely. It seemed to me that he did appreciate me speaking to him: the more questions I asked, the stronger his nod became. He seemed responsive to being informed about what we were going to do next and why. He was listening.

My patient had not been out of bed in a long, long time, which rendered him virtually immobile. He really couldn't move his limbs. When, to assess his comprehension, I asked him to squeeze my hand, I felt a small quiver in his fingers: that was his squeeze. I knew his vision was compromised; he didn't look directly at me unless I was right in front of him. I learned later that I was just a blur; it would be the sound of my voice he would remember and not my face. I had been told he was depressed—and with good reason, it seemed. Someone very close to him had died from the same disease he had, and at an early age. He knew his fate.

He had a tracheostomy (a breathing tube inserted at the front of the neck so that the mouth is free) and was intermittently on a ventilator—mostly at night, so as to allow him to rest—and he was unable to speak or write. Some patients are able to move their lips well enough to communicate full sentences. My patient was unable to do this. He had not spoken in a while.

The advantage of tracheostomies is that if we are able to successfully wean patients from the ventilator, and if they are strong enough, they will be able to speak when we put a cap on the end of the trache. The respiratory therapist (RT) assigned to my patient this particular day suggested this goal at the start of the day—so that became our plan: wouldn't it be great if our patient was strong enough to speak? We told him our plan and of course he was willing to try it. I couldn't believe it.

The moment we attached the "cork," he spoke—and then it seemed he didn't stop speaking. The difference between who he had appeared to be earlier and who he became once he spoke was startling. He was no longer an inanimate being in a bed whose thoughts and needs were unknown. He literally came to life. There was power and intelligence in his voice. It was really something to see. He had been liberated from a silent, locked-in world and helped to enter a place where he could assert himself and make himself known.

His initial words disturbed me, yet, somehow, they weren't entirely surprising. He said he felt that some of the nurses were treating him as if he were already dead. They would speak about him in the room as if he were not there and could not hear them. He said he heard sounds of disgust when they looked at him (he had an open wound that required daily packing with wet gauze; some nurses found this hard to do). He said he just wanted to be treated like a human being, like everyone else. He said his mind was alive, he could feel and hear. He wasn't stupid. He recited his social security number, his wife's social security number, their home telephone number, his cell phone number, and her cell phone number, to prove that he had a mind that could think, remember, and process information. He seemed to feel a need to prove his intelligence, to convince us that despite his inability to speak he was a thinking, feeling, living human being who just wanted to be treated with respect.

His words were disturbing and yet humbling. I wondered whether I had treated him disrespectfully. Was I guilty, along with the others? He said he didn't want to name names, he didn't want to stir up trouble, he just needed to speak it and then leave it. I told him we needed to hear this kind of feedback in order to learn and grow, and not treat other patients in that dehumanizing way. He said he understood but still didn't want to speak of it any further.

I had not thought seriously about the relationship between power and voice until that moment. It's so obvious, really: we communicate who we are primarily through our voices. If we lose this capacity, we become almost personless, we become bodies in beds, enigmatic beings. This is one reason many nurses like for their patients to have photographs in the room. The photographs are testimonies to the humanity and personhood of the patient: she did have a life before she came here, he laughed, paddled a canoe, drank wine, rode a motorcycle, hiked in the woods. . . . It is strange and unfortunate, but we can easily disregard the humanity of our patients. Their capacity to speak keeps us linked to their personhood. Their voices remind us that they are in there; they are people who command attention. Whether we like it or not, we do treat patients differently if they cannot speak.

It's awful. I cannot tell you how many times I have said to patients, "I'm sorry, but I cannot read your lips." Then they sigh in exasperation and defeat, once again locked in with whatever it was they wished to communicate, which may have been something as simple as "Could I please have a mouth swab?" or "Could I be turned to my other side?" Sometimes, when I succeed in reading their lips, I'm astounded at how simple (or complicated) their requests can be: "What time is it?"; "Where is my wife?"; "What's going on?"; "How am I doing?"; "Who are those people outside of my room?"; "My leg hurts, could you move it for me?"; "What is that doctor's name?"; "Could you turn out that bright light?"; "It's noisy in here"; "What is the weather like today?"; "Am I ever going to get out of here?"; "I feel discouraged, I want to die . . ."; "I miss my dog."

There is another aspect of this communication issue that I should perhaps mention: the connection between voice and intimacy. The relationship between nurse and patient changes when communication channels are open. When patients are able to communicate their feelings, fears, and needs to us, our relationship can become more intimate—and intimacy can be hard. It makes us feel things and can trigger our own fears of death, abandonment, loss of control. It pulls us in. There is a mystery to intimacy and I must say that sometimes I do find it very hard to look into a patient's eyes. It scares me, the intimacy scares me. I am afraid I might cry. I don't always want to see a patient's suffering and despair, and intimacy draws me in closer, to glimpse how hard it must be to lie in a bed all day wondering whether you are going to get better; or to lie in a bed waiting for death to come; or to lie in a bed not knowing who you really are and what is going on. I have sometimes felt tears well up and have had to look away, just not able to bear the feelings.

I gave a patient a popsicle once. He had been unable to take anything by mouth for many months. He had been with us for more than 100 days and had kept his strength up enough to be able to write. It was amazing to see an intact mind after such a prolonged stay. I became his favorite nurse because of the popsicle. The taste was something he had not had in such a long time. It made him so happy. It wasn't even my idea—it was the doctor's idea, but because I was the one who brought it into the room, I got the credit. This simple popsicle created a connection between us, and honestly, it was intimate. I had a hard time looking into his eyes after that: there was so much feeling there.

Just recently a patient mouthed to me that she wanted to die, please no more treatments. She had a breathing tube in her mouth, attached to a ventilator. It was very hard to read her lips but I was able, through a series of questions, to figure out why she tried to push me away every time I explained what I was going to do or what the plan for the day was. She confirmed that she did want information about what was going on, so I included her in everything we were doing. But she wanted none of it. It was so hard for me to tell her that I did take her seriously and I did want to honor what she wanted but was unable to because she was attached to that machine, which took away her voice—and if we were going to make a decision as serious as a decision to stop treatment, then we'd need to get that tube out of her throat so that we could speak about it. She was too sick to have the tube out, so we talked her into a tracheostomy. I told her it would allow her to make decisions for herself, once she was off the machine. She seemed agreeable to this, only because I was promising liberation and power.

So, even when people attempt to communicate and manage to communicate successfully, that may not be good enough. We need a sustained dialogue with people, to be able to honor their wishes. This woman did get her wish: she did die the following week, but only after we did a few more things to her that she didn't want. We did them to save her life because we were not sure if she would make a different decision if she was feeling better. How much of her wanting to die was because she was in pain and just not doing well? If we could get her better would she be glad we did? Her family members did not know her wishes (she had never been this sick before) and agreed that we needed to err on the side of preserving her life, so we did, but she suffered complications we couldn't fix and she died.

Power and voice; power and voice. I would love it if research dollars were dedicated to creating a communication device for people who cannot communicate conventionally. Stephen Hawking has a device, doesn't he? What about all of our patients lying in ICU beds around the world? I know it wouldn't be a straightforward intervention, an easily attached device that would immediately offer patients full communication capability so that they could make decisions for themselves. (I am neglecting to mention the number of patients who are confused after being in the hospital for so long. This population of patients would not be able to communicate in a meaningful way. But what about those who are capable of self-expression?)

My depressed patient did get out of the ICU. He won't be coming back: bringing him back won't help him or change his outcome. He would just end up dying on a ventilator, unable to speak in his last moments. The last time I saw him he still had the cork on his trache and was able to speak, his wife at his bedside. I still marvel at his transformation. Once he was able to speak, his wife called all his friends to come in and see him. It was fantastic. There were five or six visitors in his room. We usually allow only two visitors at a time in the ICU, but, hey, this was a special case. So they were all in there. I stayed outside the room so they could visit with him. I am not sure what he was saying that made them laugh so hard but everyone was laughing, over and over again. I thought, wow, this guy is a comedian, who knew?

He wants to live. He told us that. He asked us what kind of a chance he has. He feels technology is better now than what was available when his relative died from the disease. We didn't tell him that there is no new technology to save him from this disease. Instead we emphasized that we should work on enriching his life as best we could, now. Let's just go day to day and see what happens, let's try and get you stronger. Most importantly, perhaps: let's keep you talking; let's keep your voice alive.

Nursing the Machines

~

Cecilia Fulton, RN, BScN

"So, WHY DID YOU decide to go into nursing?"

I looked up at the face of my first nursing teacher, who was asking me that question. Many of my classmates had a long tradition of nurses in their families. Others were drawn to the profession by the prestige of starched white uniform and cap, and others were apparently just so damn caring that they never considered doing anything else. Nursing was their "calling."

"I didn't think I could make it as a professional game show contestant," I told her. That was my brilliant reason for deciding to become a nurse.

Some ten years after cracking that joke, I rose through the ranks and found myself working in the busiest ICU in one of the largest medical centers in Canada. For many years, being part of that elite group of ICU nurses felt like the place where I belonged. It had never been enough for me to be a floor nurse, working in the general medical-surgical wards.

It had taken me a while to master the technical aspect of my job, learning to operate the machines and to keep the miles of IV tubing from strangling the patient. But after a few years, after I had progressed from novice to expert, I even began to look forward to challenging, busy days when my patients were so critically ill and unstable that I barely had time to look at them, much less talk to them. Keeping fluids balanced, titrating inotropes, weaning patients off the ventilator were skills that kept my mind engaged. At times, I was so focussed on the equipment, it felt like those machines—the ventilator, cardiac monitor, drains, IV—were my patients.

I worked in the ICU for years. I progressed to teaching new medical residents and putting them through their paces. I cherished moments like witnessing a transplant recipient take his first breath with his new set of lungs. I bonded with the other ICU nurses when we went out for drinks after work and got together on our days off, swapping our ICU stories and gossiping about the indiscretions of some of our fellow nurses.

Not many of those patients made it out of the ICU; many of those who did probably didn't make it home. They were still extremely ill, many chronically so, with multiple medical problems. To me, the ICU was kind of like a game show: you never knew what was waiting behind door number one or two. . . .

It was probably a combination of age and personal growth that drew my focus from the bells and whistles and back to that person sinking between the bed rails. I am all for not going "gently into that good night," to quote the poet Dylan Thomas, but for God's sake, when that's what someone needs or wants to do (and nature tells us that the end is unavoidable), who am I to pump them full of medications, tubes, and oxygen just so it can be said they fought the good fight? I do know that there were and are many patients who are alive today thanks to the care and technological expertise they received in the ICU, but there also have been individuals upon whom much indignity of interventions and machinery was heaped, in their final days and hours. Those were the ones I wanted to help, the ones with no voice, the ones whose families "wanted everything done" when there was no hope of survival. For so many patients, continuing treatment was deemed futile, yet often at the family's insistence, we would continue with full "life support." I believed in my heart that if those patients could speak for themselves, they would be screaming out to me, begging not to be put through all this. The term "life support" became an oxymoron to me, since life seemed to be the last thing I was supporting.

It was a difficult decision, but I had to leave the ICU.

Eventually, I found my niche in community health nursing.

I recall a recent visit with Margaret, an 88-year-old widow who had been living in the same home for the past 52 years. She had had a hip replacement and was working hard at recovery and getting back on her feet. Every time I visited her, she had cookies and coffee ready for me. After I checked her vitals and her dressing, and reviewed her exercises, we sat at Margaret's kitchen table and talked. I was gratified to see her recovery, knowing I had played a part in it. Soon, she didn't need me to be her visiting nurse anymore. But even after she was no longer on my caseload I continued to think of her whenever I drove past her house. Perhaps it sounds like a visit to my granny—in some ways that's what it was. My visits with her made me feel like I was a member of her family. In our talks, as we got to know each other, she told me that she didn't want to ever go to a nursing home and definitely did not want to be put on life support. I met her son on one of my visits and we talked openly about how determined his mother was, and how he planned on carrying her out of that house in a pine box. Margaret has made her wishes known to her caregivers and family and, therefore, when the time comes she will not be admitted to the ICU but will die at home with dignity.

I have come to believe that what Dylan Thomas compels his reader to "rage against" might more appropriately be understood not as imminent death but as the loss of one's independence. For Margaret and countless others, having to give up their car, move out of their house, rely on the unreliable kindness of others is a fate worse than death. Compared with being encased in a hospital bed with the side rails up, fed through a tube by a machine, and dressed by someone who has no idea what your favorite sweater is, the arrival of "that good night" may very well be a blessing—and the ICU is, for such people, the exact opposite.

I will never regret my years working in the ICU. I look back on them as some of the most exciting years of my career and my life. Many of those memories have faded; those that remain are the ones where I really got to know the person, and maybe for an instant felt like a member of their family. (Those patients know who they are, and I thank them for the privilege.)

A lack of direction led me to nursing, all those years ago. Twenty-five years later, it appears that I do care enough to be a nurse—and I'm very glad I chose to become one.

Why I Stay

~

Karen Higgins, RN

I HAVE BEEN A critical care nurse, working in various ICUs, for almost 28 years. I graduated from nursing school when I was 21 and went to work on a regular hospital floor. Three years later I came to the ICU and have never left. I was attracted to critical care nursing because of the challenges and rewards of taking care of very sick patients in a fast-paced environment. In the ICU my nursing skills are pivotal to the patient's survival. Working in the ICU, I'm always learning new things; my role continues to evolve.

People sometimes ask me what has been the biggest change in nursing over the years, and my answer is that advancements in technology and medications have resulted in changes in the types of patient we are able to treat now. Many of the patients I care for in the ICU would not have even been alive 10 or 20 years ago. New technologies and medications have given more patients a chance to survive and live longer. The challenge for me as a nurse is that when patients come to the ICU, they are more acutely ill than ever before. The assumption is that with the developments in technology and medications there is less need for the care by a nurse, but in fact, the opposite is true. Today's patients need more care and attention from the nurse than ever before. The level of acuity has increased immensely in the ICU, and therefore on the floors as well.

Let me give some examples. On a recent shift, I was caring for two patients, both of them women in their seventies. One of these two patients had severe lung disease and pneumonia, and also was diabetic. My other patient had sepsis, a blood infection that can be deadly and affect nearly every system in the body. Both patients were fully ventilated to support their breathing, had feeding tubes for nutrition and catheters in their bladders so we could closely monitor their urine output. They also both had myriad intravenous lines, into which I had to administer complex medications. They were connected to monitors to measure their heart rate and the oxygen saturation in their blood. We're talking about millions of dollars of technology and equipment being used here. But all of it is worthless without a skilled nurse to monitor the technology and manage it based on moment-to-moment assessments of the patient's condition.

My morning started with the patient with pneumonia, and my order from the physician was to wean her off the ventilator so she could breathe on her own. But this was easier said than done. When I tried to take her off the ventilator, her heart rate began to increase, and her blood oxygenation level began to drop. She became agitated. At that point, I knew there was no way she was getting off the ventilator that day, at least not until I could get her other symptoms under control. First, I needed to lower her blood pressure and calm her anxiety. To accomplish this, I needed to sedate her and then I could more closely monitor her oxygen levels and blood pressure until she was once again stable. She was also a diabetic and I was monitoring her blood sugar level and adjusting the rate of the insulin infusion as necessary each hour. Her diabetes was so unstable because of certain drugs (such as intravenous corticosteroids) that she was receiving in the ICU.

Once I was finally able to stabilize this patient, I was able to turn my attention to my second patient, the woman with the serious blood infection. When I made my initial assessment, I found that she had spiked a fever, which is a sign of a new infection. I immediately took samples of her urine, blood, and sputum to be sent to the lab for a culture, to determine what might be growing in those specimens and, if there was a bacterial infection, which antibiotics it would be sensitive or resistant to. I called her doctor to update him on what was happening. This patient was on a number of medications, each being delivered by an intravenous line—these medications included a sedation drip and an insulin drip that I had to monitor closely in order to evaluate her reactions and titrate the medications accordingly. I had to adjust the rate of medication based on her heart rate, blood pressure, and signs of wakefulness, anxiety, and pain. When I noticed that her oxygenation level was borderline normal and that her blood pressure was slowly dropping, I immediately lowered the head of her bed to improve her cardiac output and optimize perfusion to her brain. Then I started giving her fluids (saline) through an iv line, to try to help boost her blood pressure. At the same time, I noticed that her urine output was starting to drop. I again notified the physician of the changes. The patient was not responding to the fluids I was administering so I started giving her iv medications to bring her blood pressure back up.

My entire day was spent moving between these two patients, making continual assessments and then making adjustments to their treatment in light of those assessments. All of these actions had the goal of stabilizing the patients' conditions and hopefully moving them closer to recovery.

The problem is that the whole time I'm with one patient, I'm worrying about the other patient, hoping that nothing significant has changed that I might miss while I'm out of the room. Granted, alarms will go off to alert me if something goes wrong, but the best nursing care is to be on the spot with the patient and to be able to intervene and head off problems before they occur. At this stage in my career, I can walk into a room and, just by looking at a patient, usually sense how the day is going to go and if there is going to be trouble.

These assessment skills have become second nature for an experienced nurse like me. I need them in the ICU, where a patient's health status can change suddenly. I remember one patient I cared for, a young man in his thirties. He had been sent to my ICU with a pericardial effusion, which means he had fluid built up around his heart. He was also suffering from kidney disease and was on dialysis to cleanse his blood of toxins. The night before, the patient had had a pericardial tap (this means a tube was inserted into his chest to draw out the excess fluid around his heart). When I received the patient, the tube had been removed; my job was to monitor the patient and make sure that his heart function was stabilized. The plan was to get him ready to be transferred to the floor later that day and then, a few days later, home.

It is very important to carefully monitor a patient's heart rate and blood pressure for discrepancies. You need to listen through a stethoscope for certain irregular sounds that may signal a problem. Such listening cannot be done by a machine: it takes the trained ear of a nurse who knows what to listen for. Although this patient's heart rate was fine, his blood pressure was a little low—but not in a range that typically signals a problem. He was eating on his own and he seemed to be doing well. The physicians were pleased with his progress. But I soon began to sense that something was not quite right. While he was on the dialysis machine, having the toxins removed from his blood, the dialysis nurse had periodically to adjust the machine, in order to draw fluid from the patient—and each time she attempted to draw fluid, his blood pressure dropped. This happens occasionally during dialysis, but in this particular patient's situation, it seemed to me an early warning sign that something was wrong.

Still, this is not an entirely abnormal occurrence during dialysis. When I called my report in to the physician on the phone, he gave the order for the patient to be transferred. But something just didn't sit right with me. I had cared for this patient before and knew him well. He was usually able to tolerate more fluid removal during dialysis and his blood pressure normally ran high. I had a feeling something was wrong. I couldn't point at just one thing that signaled a problem. So I went to the attending cardiologist overseeing his care—someone with whom I had worked for years—and told him, "Something is just not right with this patient." I went over my concerns and asked if we could repeat the patient's echocardiogram, just to make sure, before transferring him out. This physician knew that I was a skilled nurse with good instincts, so he agreed to do it. And when they redid the echocardiogram, they found out that in fact the patient's condition had deteriorated. Fluid was re-accumulating around his heart. My patient was rushed back into surgery within a few hours. There is a good chance that had I not intervened, this patient would have been sent out to the floor with plans to possibly discharge in the morning. He could have died.

For me, this experience is a prime example of what nursing is all about. Like air traffic controllers, we watch over our patients, making sure they remain safe and don't crash. We coordinate a multitude of activities, personnel, and traffic related to our patients. We are our patients' surveillance system. As a nurse I not only monitor my patient's condition, but also act as the pilot, delivering complex technological care on a minute-by-minute basis. I am the one person responsible for the patient's survival from the moment he or she comes into my care and for making sure that care is continuously adapted to the patient's needs.

I love being a nurse, and I love using my years of experience and skill to care for patients and their families at perhaps the most difficult time of their lives. But the expectations placed on nurses have become unrealistic. At times, the workloads are overwhelming—and worse, unsafe. I cannot be in two places at once—and as a patient's medical needs become more complex and urgent, I worry that I will not be there at a critical moment to meet a person's needs. For the last 28 years I have been my patient's last line of defense; I will continue to be that until I can no longer provide safe care.

That Deep Place Within

~

Elizabeth DiLuciano, RN

I'M A REGISTERED NURSE. For the past 19 years I've
worked 12-hour night shifts (from 7:00 P.M. to 7:00 A.M.)
in a neurosurgical ICU at a major hospital in a large city,
and for the past few years, as team leader. Many of our
patients have suffered severe trauma to the brain after a
serious accident or injury. They're in extremely unstable
condition when they arrive in our unit and they're usually unconscious.

Working with seriously ill patients, who have star-
tlingly landed, with massive trauma, in the ICU, can be
quite upsetting, but we have so many duties and responsibilities that we need to fulfill for our patient that emotions
are usually a distraction. Nevertheless, the feelings remain.

When I'm not at work I sometimes wonder where those emotions go while I'm actually on the job. The answer I've come up with is that they go underground to a deep place within myself, so that I can function professionally and stay focused on my critically ill patients' pressing needs.

In a trauma case, I work with a team that includes doctors, other nurses, the blood bank, lab technicians, waiting room attendants, security, the chaplain, and other hospital employees. The family is usually around, looking to me for answers to their many questions. Sometimes I don't have the answer to the question they really want to know: Will my loved one make it? As frenetic and complex as a patient's clinical situation is, nothing is as challenging, as demanding, and as sensitive as interacting with patients' immediate family. "Family" can mean parents, grandparents, brothers, sisters, boyfriends, girlfriends, aunts, uncles, cousins, neighbors, friends and just about anyone else who the patient wants to be included in that group.

These visitors are also frightened—even traumatized—by what has happened, and they look to me for information and emotional support. Processing information during a crisis, along with the pressure of split-second decision-making, is typically overwhelming for family members. In addition to questions involving immediate care, on my shift one of the most sensitive topics the patient's family faces is that of organ donation. As the patient's nurse, I play a crucial role in conveying information on the procedures involved. Rarely is the family prepared to have this conversation with me in the dark of night, in what may be, quite literally, their most anguished hour. Yet what I describe here is nothing more than my average night at work.

In the ICU, patients are just as critically ill at night as they are during the day. Situations are rarely stable. Patients' conditions can change dramatically in the space of a moment. I might be caring for an unstable patient, trying to titrate an inotrope to boost his blood pressure, and seconds later, be called to help with an incoming case. After entrusting care of the first patient to another nurse and delegating certain responsibilities to her or him, I'll focus on the next patient, a critical trauma from the emergency room. After a report from the ER, the new patient is placed in my care. At first, while we get everything under control (if that is even possible), my mind and body are exclusively task-oriented and I perform under strict emotional control. I don't allow my emotions to interfere with the skills I'm performing. A human being's life is in my hands. I'll remain in this state for the rest of my shift, if I have to; I have to keep my mind rational and clear.

Fortunately, there is lots of help when a fresh trauma patient arrives. Everyone arrives to lend a hand and those hands swarm over the patient, connecting monitors, changing drips, inserting new IVs and central lines, perhaps working as many as six or more IV pumps, adjusting potent medications, and taking minute-by-minute vital signs, to name but a few of the activities that are taking place. When there's a brief interlude in this flurry of activity, I do my best to bathe or at least quickly wash the patient before the arrival of the family. This entails cleaning off blood, wrapping the wounds, discarding all soiled or bloody clothing and linen, disposing of any trash or other detritus, turning down the lights, covering or closing the patient's eyes, and standing nearby to greet and comfort the arriving visitors. Sometimes I even have to catch them when they collapse in shock at the sight of their loved one's battered, swollen body connected to tubes, monitors, and machines.

Although I receive a detailed report on the patient's condition, along with a provisional prognosis before seeing the patient, nothing really prepares me for what I encounter when the patient is rolled into the room. I have cared for a 32-year-old motor vehicle accident victim who was a single parent of two children, aged two and six, whose injuries were so massive she was hardly recognizable to her family. Another patient was a 14-year-old boy with a gunshot wound to the head. He had been an honor roll student, never in trouble. For kicks one day after school, he played Russian roulette at a friend's house. His mother was out of town and unreachable, so I had the boy's older brother and sister, and an aunt, to call. Another gunshot wound patient was a 68-year-old male with a self-inflicted wound to the head. His wife waited in the company of a young couple from their neighborhood. The pair approached me to tell me that these older folks were like parents to them. I will never forget a newlywed 25-year-old man who must have stopped for a few beers on his way to meet his wife after work. Those drinks cost him his life: on his way home, he lost control of his vehicle in a tragic accident.

The initial tasks involved in settling a patient after a trauma are ideally accomplished within an hour or so, especially when I have the professional assistance of the rest of the team. When we're finally ready for the family to enter the unit, the rest of the staff clears away to give the family space to visit with the patient. The only people remaining are the patient, the family, and me. It is up to me to present and explain the situation, to counsel, teach, and comfort the family as they stand at the patient's bedside and do their best to take in this overwhelming, frightening situation—and do their best to hold themselves together.

AT SOME POINT, a doctor will apprise the family of the patient's situation. Although the family members are anxious to visit the patient, they are usually overcome with emotion when they do. Though I've established my emotional reserve for the duration, I immediately form a protective bond with my new patient. This instinct soon extends to the patient's loved ones as I prepare to meet them. I don't wish to make them wait needlessly or keep them from the room. This emotional bond will not break down throughout the patient's and family's ordeal. They look to me for answers, for calm and reassurance, so I need to be strong and steady for the family, guiding them through their grief and encouraging them in their decisions. This does not mean that my eyes won't suddenly fill with tears, or that my voice won't crack when speaking, but if I can't put my emotions aside, it becomes almost impossible for me to both care for my patient and serve the family's needs. I try to truthfully and succinctly prepare them for what they're about to see. This will be hard for them, and it's hard for me. I take them into the patient's room, and after making sure they are comfortable, I pull the bedside curtains and leave them alone with their loved one for a moment. Yet not too long—there are many tasks that can't wait.

I've now become a source of strength for this family. My support has built a trust. It's so hard to answer their questions. My honesty can seem blunt: "No, he cannot survive this injury." I say it gently, but the meaning is, of course, so harsh.

"Can I do anything for you?" I ask one teenaged girl who is weeping.

"Yes, can you just put a smile back on my brother's face?" she answers, and I have no choice but to reply, "I wish I could, more than anything else."

In such moments, I almost hate this job. But I'm needed, and that carries me through the painful times.

I'm also preoccupied with another dilemma. How will the family handle the news of their loved one being pronounced brain dead? Will organ donation be an option? The two questions must be addressed immediately. At the same time, I must allow the family time to process the news, to let it sink in, to accept their new reality, and to grieve. Each of us is different and each tragedy is unique; some people accept the reality quickly, while others take longer.

As I look out of the unit and into the waiting area, I may see many family members, but sometimes it's only a wife or a solitary friend. I consider how to broach the organ donation topic; sometimes my role is made easier, when a member of the extended family approaches me with this final gift in mind. If the family members wish to donate, or *think* they do (which is often the case), they turn to me for reassurance about their decision. I gladly provide it. I'm the nexus, the point of contact with their loved one and with the hospital; the family looks to me for not only answers, but for my continued honesty and support.

I bring the organ donation nurse to them. She discusses options and explains the process in detail. Whether they move forward with donation or not, she helps them arrive at the decision that's right for them. Many times, the nurse stays with the family through the duration of the patient's care. The sadness that donation brings breaks my heart, but the family's acceptance of me and their faith in the goodness of their decision strengthens my resolve. I "take care of" the brother, the sister, the parent, the friend. The joy of the organ recipients, their families, and loved ones is not something I'm there to experience. It simply isn't part of my role. I perform the tasks ahead of me as we prepare for donation.

My shift ends. I've talked with my coworkers, the patient's team of care providers; they are very supportive. I get in my truck—a big black truck, with big bumpers and big tires, plenty of air bags, and extra-snug seatbelts—and on the drive home my thoughts and emotions become only mine. In my internal file, I've added another case. Each one helps me learn, enables me to go on, and get ready to be there again tomorrow. Sometimes, I receive a letter from the organ donation staff, thanking me for my work and our support of the program, regardless of whether the family ultimately donated. If it did, the letter lets me know the outcome, which will help me cope with the next tough cases, where presenting the opportunity for organ donation to the family is an all-too-familiar occurrence. I'm reminded that the need that offers the greatest potential for joy also carries the greatest potential for pain: the need to share our life with someone we love.

Rescue Work

~

Tilda Shalof, RN, BScN, CNCC(c)

At times, we worry about the fate of some of our patients after they leave the ICU. We want them all to continue to receive the same close attention that we are able to offer in the ICU, but that isn't possible on the floors. The problem is, certain patients still need it.

Transferring a patient to the floor is a sign of progress: it means the patient has recovered from a crisis and is no longer in a life-threatening situation. It means the patient has stabilized and is now able to do more for him- or herself. At least, that's what it means in theory. In reality, though, many of our ICU "graduates" are still fragile. Many need a lot of complex, ongoing nursing care. The average floor patient these days is acutely ill.

Medical advances have brought about a shift: conditions that once necessitated caring for a patient in the ICU now are typically handled on the floor; in turn, a patient who used to be on the floor has likely been discharged home, to be cared for by family members or, intermittently, by a visiting nurse.

A recent innovation in some hospitals is the Critical Care Rapid Response Team. Its purpose is to follow ICU patients and make sure they are progressing on the floor. But the CCRT is a relatively new development. For many years, and in many hospitals still, some floor patients have experienced complications and have had to return to the ICU. Before the CCRRT, we frequently would transfer a patient from the ICU, give our report to the floor nurse, wish the patient and family well, say our good-byes, and walk away, trying to brush aside our lingering concerns. We had faith in our colleagues on the floor, but we also knew of their onerous patient workloads and their burdensome administrative tasks and non-nursing chores they were also expected to perform. Moreover, the floor nurses often weren't as experienced as ICU nurses and usually didn't feel as empowered as we felt.

Ironically, Mr. Abruzzi was *not* one of the patients who we were worried about. He had made extraordinary progress after a long and complicated stay in the ICU. When we sent him to the floor, we had every reason to believe he would do well. He had been critically ill but after a few weeks in our care, he was in excellent shape, joking and chatting with the nurses, taking ice chips and then enjoying the clear, homemade chicken *broda* his wife brought for him. During the six weeks he spent in the ICU almost every nurse had taken care of him. He was one of our "success stories."

His illness had started with a simple paper cut on his finger that he'd got at home. From that tiny injury, Mr. Abruzzi had developed an infection that raced through his body. It was necrotizing fascitis, also known as flesh-eating disease. Within hours the infection spread to the rest of his hand. Less than a day later, the infection—evidenced by swelling, redness, pain—had traveled right up his arm. He lost consciousness and went into septic shock. In the ICU we intubated and ventilated him, and gave him antibiotics and a then-experimental drug that has since proven very helpful in such cases of massive inflammation. He was taken to the operating room, where his now-necrotic fingers were amputated, along with part of his hand. His entire arm, neck, and part of his back were opened up, the dead tissue cut away, and the entire area flushed and cleaned of all visible infection.

I was his nurse that first night, when he returned to the ICU from the operating room. He was hypotensive; I gave him boluses of normal saline and Lactated Ringer's solution to replace not only fluid volume but also electrolytes. Later that night, as I was in the midst of titrating his inotropes to boost his blood pressure, the surgeon who had performed the debridement of the infected tissues came in to see how our patient was doing. Specifically, he was eager to have a look at his handiwork. I opened up the bandages that covered more than half of Mr. Abruzzi's body. The sight was shocking. It made me think of a slab of meat hanging in a butcher's shop window. However, it was fascinating, too: it's not often that you get to see right into a living person's body. The muscles, bones, tendons, veins, and adipose tissue were all exposed: red, pink, and yellow-marbled fat. I recoiled. It was an involuntary reaction, and I didn't take long to compose myself again—but the surgeon had a much different perspective.

"What a wound! It was bad," he said, with a gleeful expression that told me that "bad" meant "wicked good," which meant, to him, fascinating. "It was beautiful," he crowed. "Man, I tell you—work of art! We were doing sculpture in the OR."

He may well have been a budding Michelangelo, but the nurses were the Master's protégés. Every day, for the next several weeks, we each took our turn, three times a day changing the massive dressings. Each time we had to push our hands deeply into the huge cavities along his arms and into his back where the bacteria had devoured all of the flesh along the way. Each time we packed it with saline-soaked sterile gauze. During each dressing change, we could see deep into his body all the exposed tendons, veins, and arteries, the muscles and bones that had been salvageable. Within a week, the tissue surrounding those internal parts started looking pinked-up and plump. We began to have hope: if we could keep that wound perfectly clean and under the right conditions, it just might heal. For a time, we were even pouring honey into the wound, after one of our staff surgeons read a scientific report touting the healing properties of honey. (Even those nurses who were known to be uptight about tidiness and order didn't mind that the bed had become a sticky mess.) There was every indication that the infection was receding. Mr. Abruzzi's vital signs stabilized. His white count returned to normal. He was weaning off the ventilator. He was awake and aware. All signs of healing.

We got to know him. His wife came in each day and read to him from *Oggi*, an Italian newspaper, and played his favorite Caruso recordings and Italian polkas on a cassette player beside his bed, over and over again. He was still on the ventilator, but he was now trached. He was engaged in active physiotherapy to mobilize his limbs and had even started walking around the ICU.

When Mr. Abruzzi had been off the ventilator for over a week, we started him on a trache mask, which delivers a flow of humidified oxygen to the trache through the open hole, or stoma. His wounds were actually beginning to close, from deep within the narrowing gaps. We could see healthy granulation tissue, and the edges had begun to approximate. When he had been independent of the ventilator for five days straight and was able to cough up his secretions well, he no longer needed the ICU. We transferred him to the step-down unit and a few days later he went to the floor.

Less than a week later, Mr. Abruzzi went into cardiac arrest.

Late in the afternoon, I heard "Code Blue, Code Blue" on the overhead announcement system. I had just transferred my patient to a floor so I knew I'd be next in line for the new admission—if this arrest patient made it, I figured, he or she would be mine. I went to prepare the room, just in case. I never expected it to be Mr. Abruzzi.

Once again he was in septic shock but now he had, in addition, a hospital-acquired infection called *Clostridium difficile*. I gasped when I saw him, just as I had when I first met him, but this time not at the horrific sight of his wound; rather, it was the shocking condition of his whole body. The man I had cared for and come to know had become huge, his body taut with fluid, swollen with infection. I had to check his name band to be sure it was him.

"Giovanni!" I called into his ear. "Wake up! Squeeze my hand."

There was no response.

Tracy, one of my closest friends—we've worked together for years—came over to me: "The lab called. His potassium was 2.9 at 1300 hours."

"A potassium of 2.9?" I repeated. *How was that missed?* Tracy and I looked at each other, then down at Mr. Abruzzi. He was a dusky gray. His limbs were cold and mottled. He was putting out only drops of urine. His dressings were soaked with yellow drainage. The most critical problem was his hypokalemia. Serum potassium levels must be kept within a strict range, usually around 3.5 to 5.5 mEq/L. Too high or too low can cause dangerous arrhythmias. A potassium of 2.9 could definitely have lead to a cardiac arrest.

Tracy went to check the rest of the lab values on the computer while I prepared a bolus of potassium chloride, a common drug that can be lethal if administered incorrectly, but is lifesaving in circumstances like these. I asked Tracy to double-check the bolus before I gave it, as we always do, especially with powerful drugs such as potassium chloride, heparin, insulin, and others. *Twenty milliequivalents of potassium chloride is the maximum dose that may safely be given in a peripheral vein over a one-hour period,* I had memorized from the medication administration policy manual. Mr. Abruzzi needed more than that, but a larger dose requires a central vein, which the ICU doctor was preparing to insert. For the present, I had only a peripheral IV to use, to begin replacing this essential electrolyte.

Tracy scanned the rest of the lab values and called out the numbers. "His pH is 7.10 and his lactate is 7.5."

Those are terrible numbers. Mr. Abruzzi was in a serious metabolic acidosis, likely due to infection. It was probably not just in his leg, but throughout his bloodstream.

His daughter came in, sobbing. "The nurses caused this!"

I greeted her but kept my head down as I removed one of the ivs from her father's arm. It had gone interstitial, meaning it had slipped out of the vein. I didn't answer her, not only because I didn't want to incriminate my colleagues, but because I knew that a number of things had gone wrong here and many people were responsible. Also, I knew that this situation was more complicated. No, the nurses hadn't c*aused* it, but they could have *prevented* it. If things were different on the floor, nurses would have been onto this problem earlier and done something about it. Nurses could have kept this patient *safe*.

"The nurses let this happen," she said. "Why didn't they do something?"

I prodded around Mr. Abruzzi's arm, avoiding her eyes and her question. I focused on searching for a vein into which I could insert a new iv. He needed fluids and antibiotics, possibly inotropes, too, I thought, as I noted his dropping blood pressure.

"The nurses caused this, don't you agree?" She kept hounding me.

I looked up. "How did the nurses cause this?" I finally asked because that seemed to be what she wanted me to say.

"Last night I wanted to come in to see Dad, but I couldn't; I had the kids with me and everything. But I called and the nurse said he was agitated and disoriented—and that's not like Dad. I know he's almost seventy and all, but you know how sharp he is. He has all his faculties. 'What are you doing about it?' I asked the nurse. You know what she said? She said, 'I'm documenting it.' Well, good for you but what are you *doing* for my dad?"

How well I know those evasive charting terms. *M.D. notified. Problem charted.* As nurses we've all done this when we've felt helpless, or that no one was listening to us, or when we were afraid to speak up. There were so many explanations for this inertia, this passivity: entrenched hospital hierarchies, sexism, inadequate nurse-to-patient ratios, disempowered nurses, and on and on. None of them justifiable, but still, these conditions are part of the stultifying environment and harsh reality that still exists in many hospitals today.

I remembered what it was like to be a floor nurse. So many times I felt overwhelmed by the workload dumped on me. I felt voiceless and invisible. At times nurses are demeaned, even bullied, by arrogant doctors and sometimes also by fellow nurses. The hospital can be a very *inhospitable*, even *hostile*, place. You see something that worries you about a patient, but no one will listen to your concern. You have questions, but there's no one to ask. You know what the patient needs, but you can't do it; your hands are tied. You know what to do but are afraid to be wrong or challenge the doctor. You call the doctor. You wait for the doctor. You pray the doctor will listen to you, take you seriously. I knew all of these situations so well because I had been in every one of them myself, earlier in my career.

Mr. Abruzzi's daughter continued her rant; I just listened.

"They neglected him. I don't think a nurse looked in on him all day," she said.

If that is true, it is terrible and wrong, but I had done similar things—and worse—when I worked on the floor as a newbie nurse. I'd been green and scared, running from room to room, taking care of one patient and knowing I was needed by another patient. Never having a moment to sit and talk with a patient. Never able to give close, individual attention to patients, never feeling in control of my work, that it was all too much for me.

"I want answers," the daughter cried. "Why is he like this? Daddy, wake up!" She turned back to me. "Maybe here in the ICU you guys'll fix things." She tapped her foot. "God, I need a cigarette." She brushed away a tear. "This is all because of the terrible health care system we have."

I looked down at Mr. Abruzzi lying in the bed. How had he slipped through the cracks? How could so many people have dropped the ball? It was true, his complex care required the juggling of many balls at once, but so many of them had been fumbled! It seemed like all of the gains we'd made in the ICU were lost and we were right back where we started. Would we be able to fix him this time? I went over to the nurse who brought him from the floor who'd just finished her charting. Her name tag said "Melinda."

"What's it like on the floor these days?" I asked casually, an intrepid interrogator.

"Brutal," she said in exasperation. "I work casual in Cardiology, but they were short on Mr. Abruzzi's floor, Gen Surge, so they sent me relieving. I have seven patients, four fresh post-ops, all with multiple IVs and drains. One has a chest tube and three are on oxygen. Only one can get up out of bed by himself. . ."

At that moment, Tracy appeared, wheeling over a swivel chair from the nursing station for Melinda. Tracy has always had uncanny intuition. Melinda had given us a detailed and thorough report on Mr. Abruzzi when she'd brought him to the ICU—always a sign of conscientiousness—but Tracy must have sensed something was bothering this seemingly confident nurse.

"No, I can't stay," she said when she saw the chair Tracy was offering, but she sat down and burst into tears.

She won't last long, I thought. *She cares too much. This place will break her.*

"I have to get back." She stood up. "I'm fine, really." She wiped her eyes. "It's just that I'm running full tilt the whole time and everyone is too busy to help me."

"When was it noticed that Mr. Abruzzi's potassium was so low?" Tracy gently inquired. So gently, in fact, that Melinda recognized that she was friend, not foe, and readily explained. "First thing this morning, I saw it was 3.4."

"Already on the low side," Tracy noted. "So, what did you do?"

"You haven't worked on the floor in a while, have you?" Melinda said with a wry chuckle. "Most nurses don't even have time to look at lab values, but I try anyway. When I saw that low potassium, I paged the doctor. An hour later he called me back, but I was in the middle of getting a patient out of bed, so I had to call him back. It wasn't until the afternoon that I got an order to replace the potassium, but then I noticed he [Mr. Abruzzi] was on a diuretic, so I held that 'cause I knew he'd lose more potassium. I took his blood pressure and noticed it was on the low side. Then I saw his potassium pills on the bedside table. He hadn't even taken them. Maybe he was confused or forgot, but I had no time to even ask him, and then I noticed his IV wasn't running very well—I think it had gone interstitial—but by then, another call bell was ringing and I had to run off. I thought, I'll get to it later but in the meanwhile, I'd better check that potassium again, so I paged the doctor for an order to do blood work, but he was down in the ER with someone who was *really* sick. Meanwhile, a patient needed a bedpan, a family member was asking me questions, and I didn't get back to Mr. Abruzzi until he arrested. I was the one who called the Code Blue."

I returned to Mr. Abruzzi. His blood pressure was beginning to stabilize with fluids and the inotropes. An hour had passed, so now, with a central line in place, I gave more potassium chloride. I took a 12-lead electrocardiogram (or EKG), scanned it for any obvious problems, then clipped it to the chart for the doctor to review. I listened to his chest and heard crackles in the bases that concerned me. The doctor ordered an x-ray and we reviewed it together. Yes, I thought, here in the ICU, we could rescue Mr. Abruzzi. The problem was we couldn't keep him safe. We could save Mr. Abruzzi, but what about the nurses who were drowning? What lifeline could we throw them? Their affliction was not hypokalemia or sepsis, but something just as serious: fear, disillusionment—and despair.

The hospital will never be healthy for patients if it's not a healthy environment for nurses, where their voices are heard and where they can care for their patients and use the full extent of their knowledge, abilities, and skills. After all, hospitals today have become one big intensive care unit: all patients need *intensive caring.*

Conducting an Orchestra

~

Sherrill Toldy Collings, RN, BSCN

I AM A NURSE in a busy ICU in a large, urban teaching hospital. My role is called "patient care coordinator," which combines administration, management, professional development, and clinical leadership. I've been working in this ICU for the past 20 years, for many years as a bedside nurse, and now as a PCC. Even after all these years, I still love the excitement and adrenaline rush that critical care provides. Recently, I've come to view my role as that of an orchestra conductor: I bring together a variety of instruments, voices, and sounds, and I coordinate them to make beautiful, harmonious music together. Each day, I try to bring order out of chaos. I work with my "musicians," the nursing and medical staff, along with all the other members of the multidisciplinary team, to coordinate admissions, manage the flow of patients throughout the hospital, plan patient discharges and transfers, ensure that there is adequate staffing for our patients, and communicate with staff, family, and patients. I see my role as enabling the staff to give the best possible care to our patients and their families.

So many wonderful things have happened at work over the years, but for some reason, I will never forget my worst day in the ICU. Strangely, it was the most challenging, frustrating, yet also the most satisfying and rewarding day of my career.

It was a Saturday and I was training a new charge nurse that day. The day started out like any other. We sat together in the "fishbowl," a glassed-in conference room at the center of the ICU, listening to the night shift charge nurse give his morning handover report on each of the 20 patients in the ICU. We were full that day—not one empty bed. All of the patients were very ill, but a few worried us more than the others.

At that early-morning hour, everything was more or less under control. We got up and went about our daily routines. Within an hour, chaos erupted: A lung transplant patient started to deteriorate. His oxygen saturations were dropping and his blood gases showed a worsening metabolic and respiratory derangement. He was switched from conventional ventilation to high-frequency, jet ventilation. At the same time, he was in and supraventricular tachycardia, or SVT. The patient required electrical shocks, or cardioversion, many times. In fact, we needed to perform that procedure so many times to get the patient back into a normal sinus rhythm that we left the cardiac arrest cart in his room and attached to him, the paddles all ready for use as necessary.

Just before noon, a nurse came up to me with tears in her eyes. We had a death in the ICU. It was not unexpected, but it was a 45-year-old man with metastatic colon cancer. I started to help the nurse clean and prepare the patient's body for the morgue, but was called away to help care for another patient. This was a 25-year-old man whose condition was rapidly worsening: He had had a dental abscess. Although he had been started on antibiotics, the infection had tracked into his chest and around his pericardium. I saw the premature ventricular contractions on the cardiac monitor and noted how frequent and differently shaped each one was. The multifocal nature of this arrhythmia informed me that his heart was very unstable and irritable. His blood pressure was dropping rapidly and his oxygen saturations were plummeting. His nurse and I both knew he was pre-arrest. I ran to the ward clerk to have her page the thoracic surgery fellow, who had just been to see this patient on rounds. We paged stat a couple of times with no response. I pleaded with our hospital switchboard operator to break with usual policy to have this doctor paged on the overhead announcement system. (In order to cut down on ambient hospital noise, we try to limit those public announcements.) This time was an emergency. A patient's life was on the line. After a few minutes, there was still no response from the surgeon, but by now, we were running a full code. The patient had gone into cardiac arrest.

Our ICU physician called, "Sherrill! Set up the open chest tray! I'll open his chest myself." I was scared that this doctor might not have sufficient experience in doing this procedure—yet I knew it was absolutely the necessary thing to do. I was upset, too, that our young patient, a person who had previously been so healthy, was suddenly so critically ill. I knew his family was out in the waiting room, but there was so much chaos in the patient's room and the situation was still so uncertain that I didn't know what to tell them. Nonetheless, I went out to explain what was happening and to let them know that we were doing everything we could to save their son's life. I asked if they wanted to come into the ICU to be present during the arrest. This is a relatively new option that we offer to families, and in some ICUs it is still a controversial policy, but I wanted them to know they could be present if they wished. Knowing the scene going on in the ICU at that very moment would look shocking, and seeing their fragile, vulnerable emotional state, I hoped they would decline to be present for the arrest, and they did.

I returned to the ICU and went straight to their patient's room. The doctor had opened the chest and had started internal cardiac massage. The thoracic surgery senior fellow had arrived by then. Next thing we knew, I was helping to rush this man, with his chest wide open, his fibrillating heart exposed, to the operating room for emergency surgery. Off we went, rushing through the halls, three nurses, two doctors—one of whom was manually pumping the patient's heart, leaving a trail of blood in our wake—and one respiratory therapist who was delivering breaths of oxygen to the now unconscious, heavily sedated patient and protecting his airway. After making sure the patient arrived safely to the OR and seeing the surgery begin, I returned to the ICU.

The ICU doctor and I went straight to the young man's parents. The meeting was very difficult and emotional. After we left the family in the quiet room, this very tough surgeon began to sob in the hallway. I took him into my office for privacy and we debriefed with the respiratory therapist, who also was in tears. And then, in the midst of our emotional pain, we heard the strains of a mournful yet uplifting hymn, "It Is Well with My Soul." A 30-year-old woman who was dying of cancer had the song playing on her portable music player, in a nearby room. Her young husband was with her at her bedside.

I was so emotional that that soulful music seemed to take me far beyond my immediate reality. The whole day seemed so surreal, so beyond what I could cope with. I felt stretched to my limit, physically, mentally, spiritually. "No," I said to myself, "it is not well with my soul." I began to sob and a few of my nurse colleagues, with their uncanny ability to know just when I need them the most, arrived to comfort me.

Later that day, this woman passed away, her grieving husband by her side. It was the second death of the day. As I was about to help the nurse clean and prepare the dead woman's body, the OR called with the news that our young man had died on the table. I had to go and deliver this news to his parents. I went down to the OR to help bring the body back so that his parents could spend some time with him in a private room in the ICU, but I met with resistance when I got there. The OR nurse did not want to help me move the patient. She told me to send the parents down to the OR and she'd let them in to see his body. There was no way I was going to ask these grieving parents to come down to the cold, messy operating room to see their son's dead body, stretched out on the table with his chest cut open, his organs exposed, surrounded by blood-splattered equipment. I leaned in, looked into her eyes, and said, "If I have to move this boy's body all by myself, I will do that so that his parents can spend time with him in a more comfortable place, surrounded by the staff who cared for their son and who they had gotten to know." She shrugged her shoulders and went about her work.

I called for help from my own staff to move the body back to the ICU. Luckily, someone came to assist me. That was the third death of the day. If we kept this up, I was afraid we were going to set something of a strange, macabre record.

When I eventually returned to the ICU, I went to the room of the young man who had died on the operating table, to retrieve, restock, and clean the cardiac arrest cart. Meanwhile, another patient, a young woman recovering from an overdose of alcohol and Ecstasy, was showing signs of a rapid deterioration. I ran to get the other cardiac arrest cart. It was just outside the room of the lung transplant patient who had been doing so poorly that morning. I knew the nurse had left it there just in case she would need it. I looked at the cardiac monitor and noted that his heart rhythm had now stabilized. I reviewed his situation with the nurse caring for him and she informed me that indeed, her patient's condition was improving. I felt I could take a chance and disconnect the ECG leads and move the cardiac arrest cart into the room of the overdose patient, who was now in full-blown cardiac arrest.

I saw his young, scared-looking wife glance at me with a bewildered look. To her, I realized, it looked like I was removing her husband's life support. I rushed to reassure her that what I was doing was safe. "Your husband has stabilized now. He doesn't need the crash cart.

I need this for another patient in the ICU who is much sicker right now." I ran out of the room, pushing the cart ahead of me, feeling guilty at my hasty explanation.

Later, I found a moment to go back to speak with her. I wanted her to know that her husband was safe, and to understand that even in the ICU, resources are limited and we have to share them. I felt it would help her realize that although the ICU had been quite hectic that day, her husband, in contrast, was stabilized and doing very well: he had a new set of healthy lungs inside of him and his condition was looking positive.

It was late in the day and I went to check on the overdose patient who had arrested. She had been successfully resuscitated and it looked like she might make it, but it was still unknown if she had suffered any brain damage from the drugs she had taken. Her outcome was still uncertain, but for now, she was improving. I nodded at the family standing around her bed to indicate that things seemed to be going in the right direction.

Finally, my shift was done. It had been the most challenging day of my career, but I knew I had conducted the orchestra well, brought out the best in all the players, and out of chaos had made possible the best, the highest level, of patient care. Together, we had made beautiful music.

Tipping the Balance

~

Matt Nathan Castens, RN, BA, CCRN

STEVE HAD BEEN DOING everything right. He was an experienced motorcyclist heading to work on a sunny day. He was wearing a helmet. He also had the unfortunate timing of being out on the road when another motorist, returning home after a night of heavy drinking, crossed the median and hit oncoming traffic at full speed. Steve was the first person hit. Because he was wearing his helmet, his head was intact, but all four of his limbs and his pelvis were completely smashed and he suffered extensive abdominal and spinal injuries.

The crash occurred close to our facility. Steve was quickly stabilized by the paramedics and brought to our emergency department. The trauma team flew into action and completed the stabilization process, sending him to surgery to repair what internal injuries they could. They removed his spleen and part of his colon, and left his belly open to allow for the swelling that would occur. His spinal injuries, while unfortunate, did not need immediate attention, and orthopedic surgery would have to wait until he was more stable. Even though he'd been wearing a helmet, a CT scan of Steve's head showed that his brain had been severely shaken inside his skull, causing bruising and swelling, but the extent of brain damage was unknown.

His mother, Ruth, waited in the ICU family lounge throughout the long surgery and was brought in to see him when he arrived in his room. She was devastated, of course, but much calmer than we would have expected. She stroked his head, whispered in his ear words of love and encouragement, and said some heartfelt prayers. She spoke the understanding refrain of love in the face of death: "He's a strong boy. He'll pull through."

We believed that was unlikely, if not impossible. His internal injuries were massive and he'd lost a lot of blood. The orthopedic injuries were extensive and he lost even more blood from those. While his spinal cord was not severed, the location of the injury and resulting swelling indicated that Steve would never walk again. He was far too sedated for us to be able to evaluate brain function, but no one was optimistic. Assuming he did pull through, he would likely spend the rest of his life wheelchair-bound in a nursing home.

The following weeks were long and hard. With every slight improvement, Steve's family and friends were elated. With every slight decline, they told us they still believed Steve would come home.

He kept getting worse. The splenectomy had initially saved his life, but now, without that powerful organ of the immune system, infection was a constant enemy. Furthermore, while his abdominal injury started healing, problems came from other areas. Even after surgeries fixed and stabilized his broken bones, the damage from the crash destroyed enough muscle tissue to leak thick proteins into his circulatory system and severely damage his kidneys. Steve now required dialysis. The surgeries also created more avenues for infection, which had to be closely monitored. Whenever the sedation was lessened in order to evaluate his neurological status, it was clear that his brain had been damaged—although it was difficult to determine to what extent. Between the dialysis, the frequent infections, and the surgeries, it was difficult to keep his blood pressure stable, and he required multiple medications to regulate it.

At about the one-week mark, the care team started discussing the need for a tracheostomy. Steve's breathing had been supported by a mechanical ventilator. The endotracheal tube, while beneficial in the short term, was adding complicating factors: it was another route for infection, and its constant presence would, over time, damage Steve's vocal cords and trachea. In a conference with Ruth and her family, the physician and nurse presented their plan for a tracheostomy. They explained that it was no cure or guarantee, but it was one more thing we could do to help Steve's recovery.

Ruth said no.

Could that be right? Did she understand what the medical rationale was?

She said she understood, but "Stevie's a proud boy. He would never want a hole in his neck—he always believed that was a sure sign of the end."

Maybe she didn't understand the dangers of leaving a tube in the throat for a long time? Did she realize that, if the tube were left in too long, Steve might never be able to talk again?

"I understand," Ruth replied, "but I know my boy. He would not want this."

As I received this information in report that evening, I shook my head. Denial had taken over and gone from being a necessary coping mechanism to being a destructive guiding force. Who would want to have an uncomfortable tube down the throat for what would likely be many more weeks, if not months? Who would want to take the risk of being rendered alive but mute? Clearly Ruth was not facing reality—it was time for the ICU nurses to start working their stuff as patient advocates.

But Ruth came from stubborn stock. At first, she

very politely disagreed with the nurses. After several more conversations, she simply glared at us if we even broached the subject of a tracheostomy. Eventually, we gave up.

Things got worse. Infection erupted in Steve's right leg at the site of surgery. The antibiotics didn't work and the tissue became necrotic. Cultures revealed the organism was an antibiotic-resistant and highly potent infection called streptococcus A. It's what the public knows as "flesh-eating disease." It's a fast-moving infection and the only "cure" is drastic: amputation of the limb well above the site of infection. Fortunately, the site was in the foot, so perhaps Steve would only lose the leg below the knee. Ruth consented to the surgery. "Anything to help my Steve come home," she said.

Unfortunately, the operation did not help. As the infection spread, Ruth consented to more amputations— above the right knee, below the left knee, and below the left elbow. The final two most drastic surgeries she also consented to quickly: up to the right hip and up to the left shoulder. Steve was disappearing before our eyes.

As nurses, we were outraged. What were we doing to this man? A man who had been, by all accounts, a healthy, vibrant, loving son was being turned into an invalid freak by a "loving" mother who could not let go! Not only that, but her choices made sense to none of us. *Her son would rather spend his life in pieces and mute than have a damn hole in his throat? No one—no one—should be forced to live like that.* It was torture, pure and simple. *It was time to give up and let the man die with whatever shreds of dignity he could salvage.*

We started to despise Ruth. The physicians agreed with us and did their best to convince Steve's mother that all was in vain, but they still went about their duties lopping off limbs and refusing to refuse any more interventions. We were angry at the doctors.

Each time I was assigned to care for Steve, I hated what I had to do. I had gone into nursing and trauma to save what lives. I knew that wasn't always possible, but I also knew when it was *not* possible. Each time I cared for Steve, I gave him my all, stopping every once in a while to apologize in his unconscious ear for the hell I was participating in creating.

Life goes on. Eventually the infection was conquered and Steve's kidneys took over from the dialysis. As he stared out from glassy eyes, his breathing became stronger and we were able to remove the breathing tube. It had been putting pressure on his vocal cords for six weeks, but what did that matter? There wasn't enough brain left to carry on a conversation anyway. We transferred Steve out of intensive care and thanked our lucky stars: we would never have to deal with Ruth and her warped sense of reality again. Out of the picture, we could relegate Steve to that place in nurses' brains that is accessed only when angrily commiserating with other nurses over a bottle of wine. Good riddance.

Seasons change. Occasionally we would get a report about Steve from a therapist or surgeon. He was starting to wake up from his vegetative state. He was making sounds—none intelligible, but sounds, nonetheless. Physical therapy and rehab were working to help him with his wheelchair—prostheses or crutches were out of the question. We would hear these reports and shake our heads. "Hurrah!" we would gloomily think, "a success," if we could call it that.

And then Ruth came back. I could spot her from down the hall one day when working in Charge. Polite and aloof, I accepted her chocolate gift to the nurses. "Do you have a minute?" she asked, smiling. "I have someone I'd like you to meet." With that, from around the corner, came a wheelchair.

I recognized Steve immediately. Looking good for all he had been through, I couldn't help but be impressed that he could navigate an electric wheelchair so well with his one hand. He rolled up to me and held it out for a shake. As I took it, he looked me in the eye and said with a voice, clear and strong, "Thank you for all you did for me. And thank you from the bottom of my heart for not putting a hole in my throat. I can handle anything that life gives me, but that has always terrified me." He patted his wheelchair. "It's not as fast as my bike, but it's still a fun ride. It's good to be alive!"

It is a basic tenet of nursing to assume the role of patient advocate. It is the ethical duty of all nurses to speak for those in their care and to work hard to ensure that the patient's wishes are followed despite influences to the contrary, be they from physicians or family members. As Steve and Ruth walked back down the hall, I couldn't help but shake my head again. Wouldn't you know? Sometimes, families do know best. Being a nurse means being a patient advocate, but it does not mean that we always know what the patient wants. Our mistake with Steve was to assume we knew his wishes based on what ours would be.

Critical care nurses deal with death and tragedy far more often than does the average person—and more often than the average nurse. Trauma nurses also face tragic situations that many times are the result of either poor choices or poor timing. A nurse working in a trauma intensive care unit at times gets to see the worst of both worlds—but also the best. This was one of those times.

Tennis, Anyone?

~

Karen Klein, RN, BSCN

When I got to my day shift at the step-down unit, I was surprised to see Mick's wife at his bedside. In all the time he had been my patient, I had never met a member of Mick's family: they visited earlier in the day and were gone by the time I arrived on shift. I was happy to finally meet his spouse, a well-groomed woman in her early seventies.

"It's our anniversary, so I decided to stay late with him tonight," Mick's wife explained, adding, "it would have been—" She stopped herself. "It's fifty-one years today."

I gave her an understanding smile. She missed him, of course. The man she'd known and loved her whole life was, in essence, gone.

Eight long months ago, Mick walked into the hospital to have triple bypass surgery for coronary artery disease. He had already had the much less invasive coronary angioplasty, but it had not been successful, and because he was a brittle diabetic, open-heart surgery would be particularly risky for him. In fact, Mick had been refused the surgery at three other facilities but had doggedly persisted, finally locating a cardiac surgeon who would perform the operation at our hospital.

Mick did well the first two days post-op, but on the third day, he suffered a massive stroke, which left him comatose. After several weeks in the surgical ICU, Mick was able to breathe independently and was off the ventilator, and was transferred to my step-down unit. A month later he developed a severe pneumonia, and though he was treated with IV antibiotics, his respiratory status worsened and he was transferred to the medical ICU to be placed back on a ventilator.

I took care of Mick many nights during his first stay in the ICU. I watched, horrified, as, due to fluid retention, he became bloated and swollen. Eventually, when the fluid was reabsorbed, he shrunk down to a cachexic shell of the man he must once have been. I could see from the pictures his family had left at his bedside that Mick had been a tall and handsome man of 72. He sported thick, distinguished white hair and carried himself proudly.

One of Mick's biggest problems was his uncontrollable diabetes. No matter how hard we tried to regulate his blood sugars, they fluctuated wildly. We carefully monitored his liquid tube feeding intakes and monitored his blood sugars closely. This involved pricking his fingers every four hours each day, day after day. By now, months down a very hard, bumpy road through icu-land, Mick's fingers were a mess. Some were so calloused they yielded no blood at all, no matter how hard you pressed when sticking him. Others were so swollen, sore, or bruised that they were nearly unusable. Eventually I began to feel terrible, almost guilty, every time I had to do his finger sticks.

Mick remained comatose and did not respond in any meaningful way except the occasional grimace or a purposeless movement in response to a painful or uncomfortable stimulus. He was fed liquids specially formulated for diabetics via a tube down his nose into his stomach for the first few weeks, but eventually a small surgical opening was made in his abdomen and a feeding tube inserted directly into his stomach. This was how he now received nutrition. He breathed through a tracheostomy tube placed through a hole in his neck and he was connected to humidified oxygen tubing at all times. Because he was prone to pneumonias, every few hours we would have to remove the secretions that built up in his airway by passing a thin tube connected to suction down the trache tube into the upper trachea and suctioning out the sputum—a very distressing procedure for the patient as it takes away their air suddenly. A Foley catheter was inserted through his penis into his bladder to drain his urine passively, which caused him continual bouts of urinary tract infections. His arms were nearly covered with bruises—remnants of old IVs and blood draws. Though we tried to reposition him frequently in the bed, or hoist him out to a chair, Mick was thin and the skin on his left hip began to break down. Eventually, Mick developed a bedsore, a decubitus ulcer. To relieve the pressure on that ulcer we kept him off his left hip as much as possible but then the skin on his right hip and his sacrum (backside bone) began to break down and develop decubiti as well. He was, quite literally, beginning to rot away in the bed.

While caring for this patient, I often thought of Florence Nightingale's words: "The very first requirement of a hospital is that it should do the sick no harm." Most people think that the worst possible risk of an operation, illness, or injury is dying; nurses know otherwise. Nurses know that the options include not only living or dying, but also ending up in that limbo modern medicine has made possible: we can sometimes keep a person alive to a point where his or her condition might not be considered truly living. Ending up as a piece of rotting flesh in the bed; eating, breathing, and urinating via tubes; not interacting with your surroundings except for reflex reactions when procedures are performed on you or when you're turned and repositioned; stuck with needles every few hours, day after day, week after week, month after month is really not living. It's existing . . . painfully.

This was Mick's reality. To me, it seemed worse than death. My colleagues wholeheartedly agreed. Despite our personal feelings, though, we diligently kept up his care. It was so hard to see a proud man like Mick waste away like this. In fact, even as he lay comatose in the bed, trached and tube-fed, he held his head high in a very dignified manner.

I wondered what his life might have been like had he simply accepted the advice of those first three cardiac surgeons whom he had consulted about having bypass surgery. I often wondered why Mick was so adamant about having this surgery. Whatever motivated him, it must have been powerful. His life must have been so difficult that he was willing to risk ending up like this—that is, if he even knew this existence could be one of the possible outcomes. I wasn't sure he did. I'm not sure most laypeople really do. That is why advance directives are so very important. Medical science may be able to keep you alive but the real question is, what does being alive mean to you?

I wasn't present when Mick consulted the cardiac surgeon. I wondered if the surgeon, in his zeal to operate, told Mick about the risk of ending up like this, if he informed Mick in any real, substantive way. But there was no way for me to know the answers to these questions. Mick could not tell me and I had never met a family member—until now.

I took the opportunity to ask Mick's wife why he pushed so hard to have the surgery even though three other doctors had refused him. Her response was a jaw-dropper.

"We knew Mickey had heart problems; the doctors told us. But it never gave him any trouble. It's just that he couldn't play a full round of tennis without getting short of breath and having to sit down. It really bothered him. He kept saying he just wanted to be able to play a good game of tennis like he used to."

For some reason, whenever the phrase "Tennis, anyone?" comes to mind, I still think of Mick.

About two months later, Mick died from a cardiac arrest. His had been a wrenching ten-month battle in a state somewhere between life and death—a living limbo created by advanced medical technology. I suppose it could be argued that this particular patient's condition had improved: the battle was over and the suffering ended. Maybe Mick's spirit is somewhere in the afterlife, playing that good game of tennis.

Not Just the Patient

~

Gina Rybolt, RN, BSCN

I WAS AT THE DESK looking over an EKG when a patient's wife came running out to the nursing station.

"Please come quick! Someone come check on my husband!"

These can be scary words for a nurse to hear. What does it take for a concerned family member to come running for help? At times the reason is fairly benign: the patient has started coughing or says he is having pain. Other times it's that the patient, connected to all kinds of tubes and wires, is confused and trying to get out of bed. Or they're pulling on those very important tubes and wires. You never know until you get to the patient and assess the situation for yourself.

I hadn't heard any alarms; I checked the monitor and saw nothing unusual. But with ten years of ICU experience, I knew well the fundamental nursing adage that we "treat the patient, not the machines." However, the monitor was in my immediate vicinity; the patient was not. These large, lit-up screens, full of numbers, waveforms, and flashing lights, give us a snapshot of every patient's vital signs and condition. If the parameters we've set are reached, an alarm sounds. Experienced ICU nurses are able to discern which alarms are urgent and which ones aren't. Some alarms indicate an emergency; some just let us know that the oxygen probe fell off the patient's finger. A glance told me that this patient's current vital signs (pulse, blood pressure, oxygen level) were normal. However, even normal vital signs on a monitor can be misleading. So I headed into his room, right behind his wife.

"He's breathing fast, he's coughing, and his pulse is really high!"

I looked at the patient. In his mid-sixties, he was suffering from a bad pneumonia. His recovery had been rocky and he would require a ventilator to help him breathe until the infection was taken care of. Despite the ventilator's support he did look as though he was breathing too fast. The numbers on the vent confirmed this, showing that he was breathing over 40 times per minute. Looking at the monitor, I saw that his oxygen level was fine and that his heart rate was well within normal limits, at 88. So although his breathing rate was fast, his other vital signs were encouragingly stable. I turned toward the wife; she knew what I was going to say.

"Well, it was 102 a second ago!!"

"But it's okay now. And you're right, he is breathing fast. This is the second day that we've tried to wean him from the ventilator and he's not fully tolerating the lower settings. I believe he tolerated it well at first and now he's getting tired. His nurse is in with her other patient; I'll go let her know. We'll put him back on the higher settings and let him rest."

Her shoulders relaxed almost imperceptibly but then tensed up again as she looked back at her husband lying in the bed. She started wringing her hands and talking defensively. "I don't usually panic like this, it really does take a lot to . . ."

I put my hand on her shoulder as I interrupted her.

"But he's your husband." I don't know what she was expecting me to say, but it wasn't that. Her face showed a split second of surprise before her shoulders relaxed entirely. Every feature of her face showed utter and complete relief.

"Yes," she nodded. "He's my husband. Thank you for saying that."

As nurses, our focus is the patient. But we take care of the families, too.

Making Mischief in the Night

~

Janet Hale, RN

I've been a critical care nurse for 28 years and still find the ICU as fascinating as ever. However, for some time, I'd been searching for a new challenge. About a year ago I found what I was looking for—and my career got a huge jolt of energy and renewal at the same time: I made the decision to join my hospital's Critical Care Rapid Response Team. I knew my learning curve would be steep and my responsibilities great.

The Rapid Response Team is a relatively recent initiative in many medical centers. It's designed to bring the knowledge, skill, and expertise of the ICU to patients on the floor. ICU nurses are the first responders to a patient in need, wherever in the hospital that patient is. In collaboration with the rest of the ICU team, we intervene quickly; in some cases we can fix a problem in a patient's condition before it worsens. Often, we are able to avert an admission to the ICU. If we are summoned early enough, we are able to abort a cascade of worsening events and improve a patient's outcome. Sometimes, however, a patient is too unstable to be managed on the floor and does end up being brought to the ICU. Whatever the situation, if a nurse, doctor, or family member on the floor picks up on a sign that something is not quite right with the patient, we are available around the clock to respond immediately. The warning sign might be as subtle as a hunch or a vague impression or as obvious as an irregular heartbeat, drop in blood pressure, or change in level of consciousness, any of which could signal an impending cardiac or respiratory arrest.

One thing's for sure: when my beeper goes off, I know there's a patient on the floor who's getting into mischief!

I want to tell you about a recent shift I had on the Rapid Response Team.

I was called at about 3:30 A.M. about a patient whose condition was deteriorating. Mrs. Maunders was a 46-year-old woman who had end-stage liver disease as a result of a rare condition called Wilson's disease. She had been unstable for a few hours and the nursing staff was very concerned about her. It turned out they were right. When I arrived, I took one look at the patient and knew it was serious. Mrs. Maunders was sitting bolt upright in bed. Her "work of breathing" was extremely labored; her oxygen saturations were falling into the mid-70s: she was in impending respiratory arrest. I pulled my outreach cart, which is equipped with monitors, medications, and other ICU equipment, into the room and parked it beside her bed. I rolled a computer closer to take a look at her chest x-ray; there on the screen I immediately saw the likely source of Mrs. Maunders's breathing problems. She had a large pocket of fluid, likely a pleural effusion, on her right lung.

Her oxygen flow was already up to 100 percent by face mask, so delivering more oxygen to her was impossible. I knew we'd probably have to intubate her to improve her respiratory condition.

As I made these assessments, I noted another worrisome sign: her skin color was a greenish orange. I knew the color was a sign that bilirubin was building up in her system, due to her liver failure, which was worsening fast. That reminded me to check her coagulation status, which, sure enough was disrupted due to her liver dysfunction. We would have to correct her INR, or bleeding time, before we drained that fluid collection on her lung. If we tried to drain the fluid before we normalized her bleeding time, she might hemorrhage. I therefore ordered four units of fresh frozen plasma, which contains factors that decrease bleeding time, from the blood bank.

Hopefully, once the fluid was safely removed, her breathing would ease and she would no longer be dependent on the ventilator. Ultimately, if we could get her through this life-threatening event, we could stabilize her and then, hopefully, a suitable liver would become available and she could get the transplant that could save her life.

Should we send her to the step-down unit? the ICU resident asked me. There, she would be more closely monitored than she could be on the floor. Normally, this would be acceptable, but it was a short-term solution only. Luckily, I had checked out the bed and staffing situation in the ICU at the beginning of my shift, as I always do. I knew there was a patient there who had had a lung transplant a few days ago who was doing very well. It had been on a Friday the 13th, but he had told me it was the luckiest day of the year for him! He was doing remarkably well, was on "room air" with no supplemental oxygen, and was waiting for a bed in the step-down to become available. It is never pleasant to wake someone up and transfer them out to a floor in the middle of the night, but I knew that that patient was "flying right." He was stable and no longer needed the ICU—and here was a patient, desperately ill, who, in my humble opinion (those who know me know I am far from humble when expressing my opinion on such matters), did need a bed in the ICU. Yet, that patient's transfer to step-down was stalled. Nothing was happening.

It was up to me to make things happen—and fast—because Mrs. Maunders was about to arrest. She needed to be in the ICU. Let's not waste any more precious time! Let's bring this sick patient to the ICU where she can get the treatment she needs, I thought to myself. I called Mary Lou King, our nursing supervisor, who is always respectful of nurses' judgment, and asked her to get the transportation people and housekeeping to come quickly, to move and clean beds, so that I could get this mission underway, pronto!

I looked at our ICU resident. She was exhausted, having been up all that day attending to all the other of our 24 ICU patients. But she realized that we had no choice but to play musical beds in the middle of the night in order to get Mrs. Maunders into the ICU. She agreed with my assessment of the patient's condition and my decision to transfer out the other patient in order to bring Mrs. Maunders to the ICU.

When Mrs. Maunders heard she was going to be transferred to the ICU, she was relieved, but then she panicked. "Does this mean I'm dying?" she managed to say, between gasping breaths. No, I assured her, we were doing everything we could to help her.

"Is this it, am I going to die?" she repeated.

To myself, I had to admit that she might just be right. But I knew I was going to do everything I could so that wouldn't happen. What Mrs. Maunders needed at that moment was hope and something to hold on to—which, come to think of it, are probably the same thing.

"No," I said, "we're going to help you." What this patient really needed was a liver transplant, but I had no idea whether that would happen for her. "We are going to support you," I told her. "We're bringing you to the ICU so that we can help you more than we can here. We want to make sure you don't get into any more trouble." When I teased her like that, as I sometimes do with patients, her face brightened. She understood that the ICU was a sign of hope for her. I felt proud of what we could offer her in the ICU. "You're in good hands," I told her. "Our team is going to try our best to help you." She still looked worried, but took me on my word.

Now, the immediate concern was intubating her and ventilating her until we could drain the fluid in her lungs. We had to sedate her, too, so that she would be able to tolerate the intubation and ventilation—not pleasant experiences by any stretch of the imagination. While all this was happening, my beeper went off yet again; I had to move on to see another patient. I left Mrs. Maunders in the ICU, handing her over to my very capable ICU colleagues. I had no idea what the outcome would be for her but I felt satisfied that we had done everything we could to help her.

When I came in the next evening I made a "drive-by" to Mrs. Maunders' room and saw that she was resting comfortably, her daughter at her side, visiting. The ICU team had done everything I had hoped for. Mrs. Maunders was still intubated, but she was awake enough to recognize me immediately. She was so thankful and wanted to tell me how she felt. She couldn't speak because of the tube in her mouth, so she wrote a note on a scrap of paper, to tell me how thankful she was for me having saved her life.

It's hard for me to take credit for what I did. I am a part of a team and a lot of other professionals also had had a hand in her recovery, but it felt wonderful to be recognized. I knew I had done a good job and had made a huge difference in one woman's life.

I reassured Mrs. Maunders that once she left the ICU, the Critical Care Response Team would follow her through her transfer to the step-down unit, and then back onto the floor. And then, hopefully, she would go home.

An Uneasy Feeling

~

Kathy Haley, RN

I've been an ICU nurse for 21 years. For the past four years, in addition to my role as a staff nurse in a medical-surgical ICU, I have also been a member of our Critical Care Rapid Response Team. I enjoy working with this group of professionals that goes out to patients in trouble on the floors. When I'm working as the nurse on the CCRT, I am usually the first one called to assess the situation. We use our critical care skills, which we learned in the ICU, and take them out to other areas of the hospital. The "Outreach" program, as it's also called, has proven to be beneficial: we have been able to help patients on the floors and either prevent them from needing to come to the ICU or get them to the ICU sooner and treat them before things get much worse.

I remember a patient who I went to see on the medical floor. She was an elderly woman who had been admitted for an exacerbation of a long-standing respiratory illness: chronic obstructive pulmonary disease, or COPD. The Outreach team had been asked to see her for her ongoing problem of shortness of breath. We had already been following her for a couple of days when I went to see her one Friday morning. It was recorded in her chart that she was improving. She was now able to speak a full sentence without getting short of breath. The plan was to discharge her home on Monday, after the weekend. I asked her how she was feeling. She told me that she had just come from the bathroom. I could see she was short of breath from the exertion that that short trip, just a few steps from her bed, had cost her. I continued my physical assessment of her and watched her closely. I reported my findings to her nurse and to my staff physician, who was in charge of the CCRT that day.

But there was something beyond my immediate findings that was difficult to express. I had a strong feeling that something was wrong. It wasn't based on hard evidence, because her vital signs were stable and I'd found nothing amiss in her laboratory results or in my physical examination of her. Nevertheless, I felt uneasy about the plan to discharge this patient. I kept having a nagging feeling that something was wrong, that we were missing something. I've learned to trust those gut instincts.

I decided to keep this patient on my list of follow-up patients to see over the weekend. I met with the patient's daughter and explained why I was continuing to see her mother. I promised I would follow up with her mother again the next day—but later that same day, I returned with the ICU medical resident to see this patient again.

The patient still seemed stable. She had no particular complaints. She was eager to go home and the plan to discharge her home on Monday was still in place. And still, despite all of this, my uneasy feeling persisted. The next day, a Saturday morning, I went straight back to the floor. The moment I entered the patient's room, I could see she was seriously short of breath. Her color was not good. She winced in pain when I palpated her belly and at one point even doubled over with abdominal pain. The patient's family arrived and we explained that we suspected something serious was happening. We would be taking their mother to the ICU right away.

As soon as we transferred her to the ICU, she was intubated and then taken for a CT scan of her abdomen. The scan revealed that she had a small leak into her abdominal cavity caused by a perforation of her intestine. The patient was soon taken to the operating room; a few weeks later she recovered and went home.

About a year later, around Christmastime, the patient and her daughter came into the ICU to say hello. I happened to be working that day. The patient did not remember her stay in the ICU or any of the people who had cared for her. But her daughter did. She introduced me to her mother as "the person who saved your life." She explained to her mother how I had had a feeling that something was not right and how I had kept coming back to check on her. I felt both proud and humbled by what the daughter had said. It was absolutely true and I felt very fortunate for having my wealth of ICU experience and my ICU skills. I was grateful that I'd stayed alert to my feeling of unease, even when I didn't have hard evidence to back it up.

Yes, we had saved this woman's life—an entire team had worked together so efficiently and professionally to act swiftly and aggressively. Yes, we had saved this woman's life—and there's no better feeling in the world than that.

Bridge to Transplant

~

Linda McCaughey, RN, BSCN, CNCC(c)

Twenty-five years a nurse. I've never been able to come up with an adequate answer when someone asks why I chose nursing. It just drew me in. Now I believe it was my destiny, because it suits me so much. One thing I know for sure is the time has flown by. I never expected to stay so long, but here I am today, 25 years later, with not one regret.

I started nursing on a general medicine floor. After a year, although the nurse manager was very happy with my work and wanted to keep me on the floor to develop my skills there, she suggested I take the critical care course so that I could qualify to work in the ICU. I felt flattered because it was a real compliment: she saw my potential to take on even greater responsibilities and develop my career. So I applied to the ICU, and I've worked there ever since. There have been many changes over the years and lots of new things to learn—a day at work is never boring.

In the last year or so, I have been helping to bring an exciting new technology called Novalung to the ICU. It holds a great deal of promise for some of our sickest patients with lung diseases, though ICU nurses need a great deal of additional education and preparation in order to implement the new technology safely.

My first patient to benefit from Novalung was a young woman with pulmonary hypertension, a rare, very serious lung disease. Francesca was in her mid-thirties but looked far older. She was frail, malnourished, cyanotic, and gasping when she was brought to our ICU by two burly paramedics. The intense, high-pitched whistling sound of the oxygen flowing from her face mask told me that it was set at maximum flow. She was fighting for her every breath.

I took care of Francesca for a few consecutive shifts. Many patients in her situation would be angry, impatient, demanding, and difficult to deal with in some way. It's understandable. But Francesca, in her grave illness, was so soft spoken, so appreciative, so thankful just to be alive.

For the next few days she was on a high percentage and rate of oxygen, as well as FLOLAN (its generic name is epoprostenol sodium), a medication used specifically for

patients with pulmonary hypertension. It helps to vaso-
dilate the pulmonary veins, to improve oxygenation. We
administered this powerful medication through a perma-
nent IV catheter in her chest; she also had oral medications to help her maintain a decent gas exchange and
stay alive. But time was running out and her condition
was worsening.

The intensive care team and the lung transplant team
came to talk with her and her family, and outline her limited options. The treatments that we were presently using
were no longer effective. The carbon dioxide level in her
arterial blood was rapidly increasing and her oxygen level
was decreasing. She couldn't survive like this for much
longer. She, her family, and the teams decided to intubate
her and put her on a ventilator while she waited for the
call, which hopefully would come, announcing that a set
of lungs was available.

After a few days of being intubated, however, Francesca's pulmonary function had worsened so severely that
the conventional ventilator was no longer able to support
her lung function, so we had to change to a jet ventilator,
which delivers many more breaths per minute and is usually effective in keeping the lung's alveoli open so that gas
exchange can occur. But even the jet ventilator wouldn't
be able to sustain Francesca for long. The jet ventilator
would have been the last option for Francesca if she had
come to us a year earlier, but now we had something new

to offer her that just might work and buy us some more time until, hopefully, a pair of lungs would come available for transplant.

It was the mechanical device, called Novalung, that acts as a bridging device until transplant can occur. A few months earlier the lung transplant team and the ICU had started to conduct trials of this new device. The Novalung, or "iLA Membrane Ventilator," is to be used only when all other treatment modalities have failed for the patient awaiting lung transplantation. The only real solution is transplant, but this device might be able to buy her some time until a lung transplant was possible.

The Novalung is a small, white structure that is positioned outside the patient's body and takes over some of the functions of lungs. Francesca's blood would circulate through the device and then back into her body. Her own blood pressure would act as the pump. The machine is able, through the integrated membrane, to help eliminate carbon dioxide and to a small degree, improve oxygenation. It then returns the blood to the patient with the force of contractions of the patient's own blood pressure. The device not only helps the patient with carbon dioxide removal and oxygenation but also alleviates some of the stress that pulmonary hypertension was placing on Francesca's heart.

Initiating the device is no easy task. It takes a lot of coordination and a lot of medical staff and nurses. For a couple of hours, Francesca's small ICU room became a makeshift operating room. There were OR nurses, lung transplant surgeons, respirologists (also called pulmonologists), intensivists, ICU doctors, perfusionists, respiratory therapists, a hospital assistant, and a ward clerk at the desk, ready to direct and call whomever might be required. Last, but not least, I was there, right beside Francesca, monitoring her vital signs, drawing blood, giving medications, and doing everything that needs to be done. Strangely, the crowded room is always calm during this process. Everyone knows their roles; everyone has an important job today. We are united in our mission to save this patient's life.

We all congratulated one another when Francesca's artery was cannulated and the Novalung device was initiated.

Francesca stayed on this device, heavily sedated and unconscious, for six weeks—and finally the good news came that a set of lungs was available for her. The six weeks that she was on the Novalung was a very trying time for Francesca, her family, her friends, and also for the numerous team members from lung transplantation and the ICU.

Perhaps because I saw firsthand how the Novalung worked to save the life of someone who would surely have died without it, I have taken a keen interest in learning to run it and in acquiring as much knowledge as I can about this new technology. I am very enthusiastic about teaching other nurses to care for patients who are on the Novalung as a bridge to lung transplant. To an untrained eye, the Novalung appears to be a simple thing, but most of the general public, and even many within the profession, do not realize the tremendous skill, attention to detail, and knowledge that an ICU nurse must possess in order to monitor and run this device while at the same time being responsible for all other aspects of a patient's care. Because all this work has the purpose of keeping patients alive so that they can reach the goal of receiving a lung transplantation, it is a very worthwhile device indeed.

My role in taking care of Francesca included not just her medical needs. She had a family, a husband, children, a sister, and parents. They all had endless questions and needed immediate answers, constant updates, and gentle reassurance. Above all, they wanted to hear the nurse say that Francesca was going to make it. We can't always promise this, but we do our best to hold out hope.

Even when Francesca finally received a set of lungs and underwent transplantation, her battle was not over. She did not make a speedy recovery: Francesca experienced complications such as infection, bleeding, coagulation issues, kidney failure, and later, when she woke up, severe depression. Weeks were spent on her recovery, and her recovery required help from every member of the team.

Eventually Francesca went home and began to live her life again.

I actually happened to see Francesca a few months after her transplant, when she came to one of the outpatient clinics for a follow-up. It really was only when I saw her husband that I realized, to my delight and shock, the identity of the beautiful, vibrant woman standing next to him. She had such a huge smile. And then it hit me: *Oh my goodness, that's Francesca!*

Open Heart

~

Meera Rampersad Kissondath, RN, *BA, BSCN, MN*

My NAME IS Meera Rampersad Kissondath and for as long as I can remember I have wanted to be a nurse. My parents immigrated to Canada from Trinidad the summer I turned 16. I had already finished my Form 5 level of education and had sat my exams for Form 6 after only one year of additional studies, so I thought there was nothing to hold me back from entering nursing school in Canada. I was adamant that I would be going to college in the fall. I dragged my mother and my aunt, who was a nurse, to St. Joseph's Hospital in Toronto and actually spoke to the Mother Superior there. She told me in no uncertain terms that I was too young to be admitted to the nursing program; I would have to apply again when I was 18. She tried to impress upon me the fact that nursing is not a glamorous vocation (she actually used that word), that it was difficult and physically demanding work, and that it took a strong and dedicated person to look after the sick. She said if I felt strongly enough about being a nurse I should try again when I turned 18.

Well, I was mad at the world. I was mad that I had been uprooted from my home, mad that I'd been forced to leave my friends, mad that I'd been brought to this foreign country that would not even allow me to be a nurse. I was so mad that when I was forced to go back to high school, I deliberately failed science, my best subject, that fall term. I may have felt that I was prepared to be a nurse, but I was still young enough for teenage angst to get the better of me.

So, it took a little longer than I expected—but I did become a student nurse. It wasn't long into my studies that I realized I wanted to be an ICU nurse. I have now worked as a critical care nurse for the past 23 years, and I'm still going strong. Most of my experience is in cardiovascular ICU nursing.

A NUMBER OF YEARS AGO, I went back to school to get my Bachelor of Science in Nursing degree. At that time, there were some colleagues who questioned the need for nurses to have a university degree. But I believe that education is the most important criterion to finally establish nursing as a profession, not merely a "calling." These days there are numerous programs in nursing at the master's and doctoral levels, nursing chairs for research and health policy, and new roles emerging for nursing at the clinical and administrative levels. More recently, I went back to school again, to complete a master's degree in the Nurse Practitioner program at the University of Toronto. But for me, bedside nursing is the role that continues to bring me the most satisfaction. As a nurse practitioner, I plan to sustain my deep commitment to bedside nursing. Wherever this takes me, my true love remains cardiovascular nursing.

My shift starts at 7:15 A.M. at the Toronto General Hospital; by 7:30, rounds start on all the patients. Nurses are expected to present their patient; this presentation includes a short summary of the past medical history; the type of surgery and the salient highlights of the surgery; the post-operative course in the ICU, with a final plan for discharge to the floor, whether in the morning or the afternoon; and a head-to-toe assessment of the patient. The prudent nurse will use this opportunity to develop a plan for managing the post-operative course more efficiently.

At no other time is the nurse's role as patient advocate more apparent than at rounds. Let's face it, there is always a crunch for surgical beds, and the push is always on to free up those beds—but if, as a nurse, you feel your patient is not ready to be transferred to the floor, you have to say so and give your proof or rationale. No surgeon wants to put a patient at risk by transferring early, but all surgeons are aware that ICU beds are precious. As nurses, we have to support our position with information and knowledge. For a typical stable patient, my presentation may sound something like this:

Mr. John Doe is 37 years old. He had a STEMI [ST wave myocardial infarction] one month ago and now has an LV [left ventricular] function of two out of four. His past medical history includes high cholesterol, smoking, and a positive family history of heart disease. Yesterday afternoon he had a CABG [coronary artery bypass graft]. . . . Surgery was uneventful and he was admitted to the ICU at 1600 hours and extubated at 1900 hrs. He's in a positive six liter balance; his K+ [potassium] and Mg+ [magnesium] have been replaced. All other chemistries are normal. Hemoglobin is 89 and INR is 1.0—all within normal post-op range. Blood pressure is 110 on 80, but filling pressures were low, so he received 500 cc of Pentaspan. Cardiac output has improved and is now 4.5 liters per minute. CVP [central venous pressure] is 10 mmgHg. He's in sinus rhythm with a rate of 90 beats per minute with no ectopics. Overnight he had a few runs of svt [superventricular tachycardiac] at a rate of 120 per minute. May need to be restarted on a small dose of beta blocker. Chest tube drainage is minimal. Plan to pull them out once he is mobilized, if all goes well. Neurologically, he is fully awake with no deficits. Respiratory condition is stable, now on nasal prongs at 4 liters per minute, O_2 saturation is 95 percent. Air entry is decreased to bases with bilateral crackles; will need Lasix. He's tolerating clear fluids and his urine output is between 40 and 60 cc per hour. The plan is for him to be transferred to the floor this afternoon.

An icu nurse is expected to present the patient and a plan of care for the shift ahead. The icu's ability to fulfill the expected surgical caseload for that day depends, in part, on the ability of the nurse to present a realistic plan for the patient. At the end of rounds, it can be estimated how many surgeries can safely be performed that day. Therefore, the purpose of rounds is twofold: to assess and manage patients' post-operative course, and to control patient flow.

At first, I found it challenging to organize my thoughts and communicate them precisely during rounds, but I worked hard on that skill. I didn't want, on rounds, to be fumbling around, hesitating, or flipping back and forth in the patient's flowchart to find the information I needed to present. I started out by simply memorizing the information, because I did not want to look foolish, but later I realized that for me it was a matter of professional pride that my presentation be informative and succinct.

A recent experience has confirmed again for me why I love working in the cv-icu. My patient was a woman in her late fifties who had had a CABG and had been extubated during the night, about six hours after her admission to the ICU. She had been nauseated so was given Gravol and was now a bit sleepy—a common side effect of the drug. After I received the night nurse's report, I delayed performing my initial assessment, in order to let my patient sleep. It's amazing how much a nurse is able to assess before laying a hand on a patient. I was able to measure her cardiac output, analyze her heart rhythm, and take her vital signs. I checked that the medications that she was on were the exact medications she was actually receiving, and I reviewed what ivs she had and checked that they were patent. After noting that her urine output was adequate, I reviewed her laboratory results from the blood sample taken during the night. I observed that her breathing was shallow, but that is common after cardiac surgery with four chest tubes in the mediastinum and surrounding the lungs.

One thing that did concern me was that the chest tube drainage for the previous hour was more than normal. Sometimes chest tubes will dump a large amount of blood when the patient is mobilized, and they may continue to dump larger-than-expected volumes for up to an hour or so later, but this patient had not yet ambulated. Also, the chest tubes draining the blood felt heavy in my hands and the blood in the chest tube drainage system had a certain thick look that concerned me. I decided to run some tests on the patient's hematological profile (such as a complete blood count, or CBC) and her coagulation function (such as PT/PTT and INR) so that I could get a more accurate picture of the clotting status and hemoglobin level. I also sent a sample of arterial blood for blood gas analysis.

By this time, my patient was awake, so I introduced myself and explained that I was going to be her nurse for the day. I told her she was doing really well and that her surgery had gone well. I continued with my initial assessment and moved on to listening to her heart and chest sounds. Since her nausea had still not abated, I decided to give her something stronger. She held my hand and tried to smile at me while the drug took effect. By then the team had arrived on rounds. I presented my patient and my concerns about the chest tube losses and told them that I had repeated the blood work. My plan was to mobilize the patient after her nausea had subsided, just in case there was a stubborn pocket of blood sitting there in the mediastinum.

She had a good sense of humor: she asked if we'd talked about her during rounds. I said, yes, that we'd been planning her care. "Well, I should feel like a star, then!" I told her she was indeed a star, that I was sorry she was feeling so poorly from the nausea, but soon the medication would take effect. Abruptly, she sat up in bed, clutched my hand, and coughed. Then all hell broke loose.

Her eyes rolled back and she fell back onto the bed. Her momentum took me forward with her. I whipped back the bed linen to see bright red blood pouring out of her bilateral chest tubes, filling the collection canister at an alarming rate. I called for help. I reached over and opened up her peripheral IV, which, luckily, had a large bore—18 gauge. I opened up her central venous line too, the one that is situated in the large neck vein. I was trying desperately to get fluids into her before she went into hypovolemic shock from the massive blood loss. I looked at the cardiac monitor and saw a rhythm, but I could feel no pulse, so I climbed up on her bed and started CPR. By then, people were barreling into the room, pushing the crash cart in and yelling out orders, asking for explanations of what happened.

"Who's the surgeon?"

"Call the surgeon!"

"Call blood bank—we need blood!"

"How many units?"

"Lots!"

"Where's the RT?! We need to intubate, right now!"

"Open all the lines!"

We pushed epi again and again and again, to try to kick-start her heart. There was still no rhythm.

"Continue chest compressions!"

"Call The Team!" In a CV-ICU there is the ICU team and then there is The Team. The latter comprises the individuals who work in the OR with the cardiovascular surgeon: cardiac OR nurses, perfusionists, and many others. They came, bringing with them the equipment they would need to perform cardiac surgery right in the room. I figured this was likely a precipitous tamponade, which is a compression of the heart due to a collection of blood in the pericerdium, most probably due to a ruptured graft. There was no time to get the patient to the OR; the OR would have to be brought to the patient. Her chest would be opened right there in the room.

Within minutes, everyone arrived. The patient was prepped and the chest sutures were cut. The chest wall was peeled back and held open by large steel clamps called retractors, to reveal a quivering heart bathed in a sea of blood. Someone reached in and gently squeezed the heart, waited for its own intrinsic electrical conduction system to take over . . . but nothing. The blood was quickly suctioned away and the area was washed and kept reasonably free of blood by a constant flow of fluid so that the surgeon could identify the rupture and re-suture the graft. While all this was going on, powerful medications were being prepared and IV drips were hung. I was drawing up drugs and sending off blood work. By this time, the activity in the room reverberated like a low hum: in these situations, the urgency is palpable but it is tempered by steely determination and purpose.

All hands were on board—this was a team, and despite the crisis and seeming pandemonium, there was order to this chaos. No one needs to be told to tie up a gown, open a sterile package, pour the chlorhexidine: things get done. Everyone knows what to do. A code or an emergency surgery like this is an exquisitely choreographed dance among many skilled professionals who know and respect one another's roles and who depend on every other dancer to get it right. Everyone knows that the life of this patient hangs in the balance.

Finally the rupture was sutured and sterile internal defibrillation paddles were applied to the ominously still heart.

"All clear?" Once. Nothing.

"All clear?" Twice. Still nothing.

The heart was squeezed gently again and this time there was no blood flow from the coronary vessels. We needed to get the heart going on its own—immediately.

Suddenly, there was a little movement. More drugs

were pushed. I stood off to the side and watched and prayed for her heart to respond.

"We've got a heartbeat!"

Yup, and a blood pressure, too, although it required support from a slew of drugs, including epinephrine, Levophed, vasopressin, dopamine, and others. Blood and plasma were being pumped into the patient; the lines were wide open. Someone was shooting cardiac outputs, sending off blood work, analyzing arterial blood gases, and making adjustments on the ventilator. She was still unconscious, but I did what I always do with my patients, regardless of their state of awareness: I talked to her, encouraged her, told her to hang on.

She was still so critically ill, we didn't know if she'd make it. Would the chest be closed? What's her lactate? Where's the family? Have they been notified?

Then came the hard part: getting this patient through the next 12 hours. There were so many immediate tasks to do that I couldn't even allow myself to think of the possible complications that might result from this catastrophe. Due to such prolonged and profound hypotension, her kidneys might not have received adequate perfusion, so she might develop something called "acute tubular necrosis." That might mean dialysis, either temporarily or permanently. Depending on the condition of her heart, a balloon pump might be added, to assist perfusion. My goal for the next few hours and the next day, when I returned to care for her again, was to help her become stabilized.

Surprisingly enough, this patient survived—that in itself is a miracle. Open-heart procedures in the ICU setting are uncommon, and when you consider the uncontrolled environment, the length of time without a heartbeat, and the patient's age, among other variables, you realize that this patient's resilience—the human body's resilience—is truly a marvel.

IT WAS A YEAR OR TWO LATER, a Monday, around 9:00 in the morning. Everyone had descended on Hospital Row, as this stretch of University Avenue in downtown Toronto is called, as the workweek began. I had gone to the first floor for a cup of Tim Horton's coffee and stepped into the crowded elevator to find that the button for each floor had been pressed, lighting up the panel like a veritable Christmas tree. The doors closed, and lulled by the muted sound of conversation, I retreated into my own thoughts. My day had started almost two hours earlier, when a real hospital day starts. The elevator door opened and closed.

"There you are! I knew one day I would see you again," a voice said.

A tiny woman stood in front of me, looking at me; I looked behind me to see who she was talking to. I didn't know this woman.

"You may not remember me, but you were my nurse when I had my surgery."

I opened my mouth to say something, but what could I say? I didn't remember her, and I was embarrassed at being singled out. The crowded elevator had fallen silent, as all eyes turned onto this unfolding tableau.

"I had heart surgery," she said, as if she were telling me she'd had mango ice cream, and it tasted good.

"Oh, yes . . ." I said uncertainly.

"And I had another attack and they opened me up right in the room. I almost died."

Now I remembered, and along with everyone else in the elevator, I became caught up in the story this little dynamo of a woman was spinning. I was so entranced by her obvious delight at being alive and her lack of constraint in the telling of this tale.

"And as I was going in and out of consciousness, at one point you said to me, 'Hang on, sweetheart, I've got you.' Your face was the last thing I saw just before I blacked out."

By then, I was so choked up I could barely speak. She reached into her bag.

"When I left the hospital, I bought this because it reminded me of you; I always keep it with me." She pulled out this blond, blue-eyed angel from her bag and took my face between her hands, pressing the pale doll onto my dark-skinned cheek. I had to chuckle at that image, but I was very grateful for her sincere intention.

"I will always remember you," she said and stepped from the elevator.

The elevator doors closed.

How can you beat that feeling? I was on top of the world!

"That would make my day," I heard someone say from the back of the elevator.

I stepped from the elevator, tears rolling down my cheeks. I felt so touched and humbled, and so appreciative of my profession. Nursing reminds me, each day, to care—in the midst of chaos and imminent death.

I have been blessed in my choice of career.

Acknowledgment of Permissions

"Intensive Care" is excerpted from *Intensive Care: The Story of a Nurse*, copyright © 1987 by Echo Heron. Published by Ballantine Books.

About the Editor

TILDA SHALOF is a staff nurse in the Medical-Surgical Intensive Care Unit at Toronto General Hospital of the University Health Network and has been there since 1987. She graduated from the University of Toronto, Faculty of Nursing back in 1983 and has worked in hospitals in New York City, Tel Aviv, and for the past 23 years in Toronto. In 1990, she achieved certification as a specialist in Critical Care Nursing from the Canadian Nurses' Association.

In 2004, Tilda published *A Nurse's Story*, a memoir of her career as a critical care nurse. It received wide critical acclaim, became a national bestseller, and has been translated into Chinese, French, Japanese, and Vietnamese. In 2007, Tilda released *The Making of a Nurse*, in which she charts the educational, intellectual, emotional, and spiritual steps in her journey of becoming a nurse. In it, she shares some of the professional and personal challenges she's faced in becoming the nurse she aspired to be. Her latest book, *Camp Nurse—My Adventures at Summer Camp* is a fond remembrance of six summers working at a variety of residential summer camps for children in Ontario, Canada. Written from the perspective of both parent and professional, it describes the joys of camp, its many benefits to children, and the ways that a camp nurse helps keep campers—and their counselors—safe and healthy.

In addition to being a critical care nurse and bestselling author, Tilda is also a frequent media commentator, a nurse and patient advocate (she believes the two roles go hand-in-hand), and an inspiring and dynamic public speaker. Her presentations include insider stories from her long career as a critical care nurse and observations about the realities of clinical practice in today's healthcare environment. Tilda addresses a broad range of audiences, but her messages resonate most strongly with frontline caregivers, both professional and lay, nurses and doctors and all other healthcare roles, specialties, levels of experience, and practice settings. She is passionate about helping caregivers re-connect with their ideals, to inspiring them to excellence in their practice, and to reminding us all about the privilege it is to do this work. Tilda is dedicated to explaining nursing and healthcare to the public and to raising the awareness of the central role of nurses in ensuring the public's health and safety.

Tilda lives with her husband, Ivan Lewis, and their sons, Harry and Max, in Toronto, Canada, and can be reached through her website www.NurseTilda.com.

About the Contributors

DR. JUDY BOYCHUK DUCHSCHER RN, BScN, MN, PhD, became a nurse in 1979 and went on to achieve a Post-Graduate Diploma in Intensive Care Nursing from the University of Manitoba, a diploma in Cardiovascular Nursing from Stanford University in California, and Critical Care certification (CCRN) from the American Association of Critical Care Nursing. Boychuk Duchscher helped initiate the heart and heart-lung transplant program at the University of Alberta Hospital, developed the multi-organ donor referral program at Toronto General Hospital, and managed the lung transplant program at Barnes Hospital in St. Louis, Missouri. She has taught at the University of Saskatchewan and holds academic positions with universities in Alberta, Calgary, and Western Sydney in Australia. In 2006, Boychuk Duchscher launched a non-profit organization called "Nursing the Future," an initiative that serves as a bridge between the ideals of nursing education and the realities of professional practice. As a scholar, Boychuk Duchscher has published widely on the topic of new graduate transition in peer-reviewed articles and book chapters. Boychuk Duchscher is a much-sought-after speaker on the topic of the contemporary climate of acute-care nursing, new graduate transition to professional practice, and multi-generational nurses in the workplace.

SARAH BURNS, RN, BScN, is a graduate of Northern Michigan University's Nursing Program. She has worked at hospitals in Massachusetts, Michigan, and Texas. Currently she works in a medical intensive care unit at the University of Michigan Hospital.

MATT NATHAN CASTENS, RN, BA, CCRN, discovered that nursing was more fulfilling than his previous career as an actor when he started working as a nursing assistant in critical care. Matthew has since worked as a staff nurse in a cardiovascular ICU, in a trauma-neuro ICU, and as a flight nurse. He now enjoys nursing staff development as the Resource Educator for Critical Care at North Memorial Medical Center, a Level I Trauma Center in Robbinsdale, Minnesota.

ELIZABETH DiLUCIANO, RN, lives in Virginia Beach, Virginia, with her husband, Gregory. She's worked in a Level 1 Trauma Hospital as a bedside nurse in a Neuro Intensive Care Unit since 1990.

CECILIA FULTON, RN, BScN. A graduate of George Brown College, Ontario, Canada, Cecilia went on to complete a Bachelor of Science in Nursing from Ryerson University, graduating as class Valedictorian. She began a master's degree at the University of Toronto but "found the disconnect between the curriculum and clinical practice to be too large an abyss to bridge." Fulton has worked as a community nurse and vows never to relinquish her nursing license. "I worked too hard to get it," she says, though in 2004, she took her real estate license. "Nursing is no longer my primary profession these days. Living in Toronto with my husband, Larry, and raising our three children is now my priority. At times, I miss the excitement of the ICU, but get discouraged when I hear that my colleagues are still battling some of the same issues we faced years ago. I am proud of them for having the energy, skill, and compassion to continue doing one of the most demanding jobs in the world."

JANET HALE, RN, graduated from Seneca School of Nursing in 1975. She worked in General Surgery, then became a critical care nurse and has worked in the Medical-Surgical ICU at Toronto General Hospital for over 24 years. "I am married to Dan and we have two wonderful daughters, Karen and Julie, but I am owned by a Scottish Terrier and three West Highland Terriers. I love to sew, quilt, knit, read the classics, such as the works of Thomas Hardy and Jane Austen. I volunteer with Team Captain of the Medical Team for the Annual Weekend to End Breast Cancer and the Ride to Conquer Cancer. . . . Life is never dull."

KATHY HALEY, RN, has worked at Toronto General for 24 years, most of them in the Medical-Surgical ICU. She has been a member of the Critical Care Outreach Team since it began in 2005. Kathy is married to Bob and they have two sons, Christopher and Connor.

ECHO HERON, RN, worked in ER and Coronary Care in the San Francisco Bay Area for 18 years. She is the author of the bestselling *Intensive Care: the Story of a Nurse, Condition Critical: the Story of a Nurse Continues, Tending Lives: Nurses on the Medical Front, Mercy,* and the Adele Monsarrat R.N. medical mystery series, *Pulse, Panic, Paradox,* and *Fatal Diagnosis.* Ms. Heron continues to champion nurses and pursue her literary career. Find out more about Ms. Heron's work at www.echoheron.com.

BOB HICKS, RN, BScN, BHSc, has studied at the University of Western Ontario (2002) and the University of Toronto. He co-authored the *Preceptorship Resource Kit,* published by the Registered Nurses' Association of Ontario. Bob currently works at New York-Presbyterian Hospital in the Surgical ICU.

KAREN HIGGINS, RN, has more than 33 years nursing experience as a front-line caregiver and staff nurse. She is also past-President of the Massachusetts Nurses' Association. During her tenure Higgins led MNA's fight to improve the quality and safety of patient care in Massachusetts' healthcare facilities, worked to increase access to healthcare for all citizens, and chaired a task force to address the nursing shortage. Higgins is a leading figure in the American Association of Registered Nurses. She currently works as a staff nurse in the Cardiac Care Intensive Care Unit at Boston Medical Center.

LISA HUNTINGTON, RN, graduated from St. Rita Hospital School of Nursing in Sydney, Nova Scotia, in 1983. She began her nursing career in Moose Factory, Ontario, a tiny Cree community in James Bay. She has worked in the ICUs at Northwestern Hospital in Toronto, Toronto General Hospital, and in Townsville, Australia. Presently, Lisa works in Medical Imaging, where her critical care skills are invaluable.

CHRIS KEBBEL, RN, BScN, is a critical care nurse with over ten years of bedside experience in the Medical/ Surgical ICU at Toronto General Hospital. He now divides his time between clinical practice and his own healthcare informatics consulting firm, Cecktor Limited, which provides clinical information systems and web solutions to healthcare clients. He can be reached at his company's website, http://www.cecktor.com.

KAREN KLEIN, RN, BScN, obtained her nursing degree from Adelphi University, graduating magna cum laude. Her varied experience includes ER/Trauma, Pediatrics, Interventional Radiology, Telemetry, ICU, Home Infusion, and Occupational Health. She is a certified Emergency Nurse, an American Heart Association CPR/First Aid Instructor and has been published by *Nursing Spectrum Magazine.*

DR. ROSEMARY KOHR is an Advanced Practice Nurse in Acute Care Medicine, London Health Sciences Centre, London, Ontario, where she has worked for 15 years. She is a wound care consultant and educator in acute, community, and long-term care settings. Rosemary completed a BA in Visual Arts from the University of Ottawa, BScN from Laurentian University, a MScN from the University of Western Ontario, and a PhD from the University of Alberta. She holds a post-Masters' Acute Care Nurse Practitioner (ACNP) certificate (University of Western Ontario) and has academic appointments in the Faculty of Health Sciences at UWO and Athabasca University in Alberta, Canada.

DR. LINDA L. LINDEKE, PhD, RN, CNP, graduated from the University of Alberta, Canada, and received master's and PHD degrees from the University of Minnesota. She is a pediatric nurse practitioner, working in educational settings as well as with infants born prematurely and their families. Her interests include health policy, children with special healthcare needs, and barriers to nursing practice. She is the national president of NAPNAP, the 7,000-member National Association of Pediatric Nurse Practitioners.

MARY MALONE-RYAN, RN, BN, studied nursing at Dalhousie University of Halifax, Nova Scotia, in 1987. She worked in General Medicine and the Medical ICU at Toronto General Hospital until moving to Hickory, North Carolina, where she works at the Frye Regional Medical Center in the cardiovascular ICU. Mary is married to Frank and they have Molly, Caileigh, and Luke Malone.

LINDA McCAUGHEY, RN, BScN, CNCC (c), has worked in the ICU for the past 24 years and has achieved certification as a critical care nurse from the Canadian Nurses' Association. Linda has helped initiate and develop the Critical Care Rapid Response Team. "Of all that I have done in the hospital, I am most proud of being a bedside nurse, caring for patients. It's not always given enough credit, nor is it the most popular choice for newer nurses, but it's what gives me the greatest satisfaction." Linda has been married to Dan for the past wonderful 25 years and they have three children, Kirsten, Shannon, and Alison.

Kirsten and Shannon are in their second year studying nursing and Alison is in grade school.

BELLA MEDEIROS MANOS, RN, graduated from George Brown College in Toronto in 1988 and has been nursing for 22 years in General Surgery, Trauma and the Medical Surgical Intensive Care at Toronto General Hospital of the University Health Network. She lives in Newmarket, Ontario, with husband Nick and their three children, William, Madeline, and Emma.

MADELEINE MYSKO, RN, MA, teaches creative writing in the Advanced Academic Programs of the Johns Hopkins University. She also coordinates the "Reflections" column for *American Journal of Nursing*. Her work, both poetry and prose, has appeared in *The Hudson Review, Shenandoah, Bellevue Literary Review, The Baltimore Sun, American Journal of Nursing*, and elsewhere. Her first novel, based on her experiences as an army nurse on the burn ward, is *Bringing Vincent Home* (Austin, Tex.: Plain View Press, 2007).

MEERA RAMPERSAD KISSONDATH, RN, BA, BScN, MN, graduated from Ryerson University (1983), McMaster University (1989), and the University of Toronto (1981 and 2007). Her master's degree has a focus on cardiology and interventional cardiovascular surgery. Meera has been a staff nurse for 17 years in the CVICU at the University Health Network and staff nurse and Nurse Clinician, Cardiology at the Humber River Regional Hospital, Ontario. She is presently working toward board certification as a Nurse Practitioner. Meera lives in Ontario with her three sons and two dogs.

SHARON REYNOLDS, RN, BScN, has been an ICU nurse for 17 years.

GINA RYBOLT, RN, BScN, graduated from Bradley University in 1997. She has worked in medical/surgical and inpatient dialysis nursing, but the majority of her career has been in critical care. Gina is the author of *Codeblog: Tales of a Nurse,* a weblog started in 2002 specifically geared toward nursing and healthcare experiences. Along with writing about her own professional experiences, Gina posts stories submitted by other nurses, doctors, patients, and paramedics. *Codeblog* has been mentioned in *Newsweek, Nurseweek, The Wall Street Journal, Proto Magazine,* and was included in the *Forbes* Best of the Web medical blogs list. Gina lives and works in California.

CLAIRE THOMAS, RN, BScN, studied at John Abbott College in Montreal and completed her bachelors degree at the University of British Columbia (2004). She has practiced in Vancouver, Montreal, and Toronto, in a variety of clinical settings. She specialized in Critical Care Nursing in 2001 and has been working in that specialty ever since.

SHERRILL TOLDY COLLINGS, RN, BScN, graduated from the University of Toronto in 1985 and has been working in the Medical-Surgical Intensive Care Unit in a university-affiliated teaching hospital in Toronto for the past 20 years. For the past 12 years she's been a Patient Care Coordinator, a clinical leadership role to support front-line staff and their patients. She completed a Clinical Manager Program at the Schulich School of Business at York University in Toronto. Sherrill lives in Oakville, Ontario, with her three sons, Matthew, Ethan and Rhys.